T0255027

Professional Practice Models in Nursing

Joanne R. Duffy, PhD, RN, FAAN, is an adjunct professor at the Indiana University School of Nursing, Indianapolis, Indiana, and executive vice president and senior consultant at QualiCare in Winchester, Virginia. Dr. Duffy's extensive career encompasses clinical, administrative, and academic roles. She has directed four graduate nursing educational programs, and has been a department chair, interim associate dean for research, and, most recently, a named endowed evidence-based practice and research professor. Dr. Duffy has held various administrative positions directing medical, rehabilitation, critical care, emergency, and transplantation nursing services at both community and academic medical centers. She also directed a nurse-led center for outcomes analysis, dedicated to improving the quality of cardiovascular services. She was a cardiovascular clinical nurse specialist with clinical experience in critical care and emergency nursing. Dr. Duffy has published extensively across the nursing literature, but is best known for her work in maximizing patient outcomes. She was the first to link nurse caring to patient outcomes, and has designed and tested multiple versions of the Caring Assessment Tool (CAT). She developed the Quality-Caring Model©, a middle-range theory used in more than 45 U.S. health systems.

Dr. Duffy was the recipient and principal investigator for two federally funded demonstration projects: *Relationship-Centered Caring in Acute Care and Improving Safety* and *Quality in Vulnerable Acute Care Patients Through Interprofessional Collaborative Practice*, and has been the principal investigator on externally funded studies of hospitalized older adults, those with heart failure, tool development, nurses' caring competencies, evidence-based practice, and academic–service partnerships. She has also consulted on studies related to organizational leadership and management of critical care units, patients' perceptions of safety, health literacy, and alarm safety. Dr. Duffy was a consultant to the American Nurses Association (ANA) in the development and implementation of the National Database of Nursing Quality Indicators (NDNQI), and was the former chair of the National League for Nursing's (NLN) Nursing Educational Research Advisory Council. Dr. Duffy is the author of numerous publications, including two books and several book chapters. Her book *Quality Caring in Nursing: Applying Theory to Clinical Practice, Education, and Research* received the American Journal of Nursing (AJN) Book-of-the-Year award in 2009. She is a former Commonwealth Fund Executive Nurse Fellow, a recipient of several nursing awards, a fellow of the American Academy of Nursing, and she serves on several editorial review boards. Dr. Duffy currently teaches graduate-level nursing research and data analysis for clinical and administrative decision making; regularly consults with health systems regarding evidence-based practice, research, and professional practice model integration; and is a frequent guest speaker.

Professional Practice Models in Nursing

Successful Health System Integration

Joanne R. Duffy, PhD, RN, FAAN

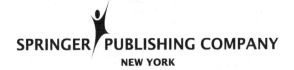

SPRINGER PUBLISHING COMPANY
NEW YORK

Springer Publishing Company, LLC
11 West 42nd Street
New York, NY 10036
www.springerpub.com

Acquisitions Editor: Joseph Morita
Production Editor: Kris Parrish
Composition: Exeter Premedia Services Private Ltd.

ISBN: 978-0-8261-2643-6
e-book ISBN: 978-0-8261-2644-3

16 17 18 19 20/ 5 4 3 2 1

The author and the publisher of this Work have made every effort to use sources believed to be reliable to provide information that is accurate and compatible with the standards generally accepted at the time of publication. Because medical science is continually advancing, our knowledge base continues to expand. Therefore, as new information becomes available, changes in procedures become necessary. We recommend that the reader always consult current research and specific institutional policies before performing any clinical procedure. The author and publisher shall not be liable for any special, consequential, or exemplary damages resulting, in whole or in part, from the readers' use of, or reliance on, the information contained in this book. The publisher has no responsibility for the persistence or accuracy of URLs for external or third-party Internet websites referred to in this publication and does not guarantee that any content on such websites is, or will remain, accurate or appropriate.

Library of Congress Cataloging-in-Publication Data

Names: Duffy, Joanne R.
Title: Professional practice models in nursing : successful health system
    integration / Joanne R. Duffy.
Description: New York, NY : Springer Publishing Company, LLC, [2016] |
    Includes bibliographical references.
Identifiers: LCCN 2015032250| ISBN 9780826126436 | ISBN 9780826126443 (e-book)
Subjects: | MESH: Models, Nursing. | Nurse Administrators. |
    Nursing—organization & administration.
Classification: LCC RT89 | NLM WY 20.5 | DDC 362.17/3068—dc23
LC record available at http://lccn.loc.gov/2015032250

Printed in the United States of America by McNaughton & Gunn.

Contents

Contributors ix
Foreword Karen S. Hill, DNP, RN, NEA-BC, FACHE, FAAN *xi*
Foreword Linda Burnes Bolton, DrPH, RN, FAAN *xiii*
Foreword Karen Cox, PhD, RN, FACHE, FAAN *xv*
Preface *xix*
Acknowledgments *xxv*

PART I. FROM AWARENESS TO COMMITMENT

1. Professional Practice Models: Raising Awareness *3*

    Learning From the Field: What Are Professional
    Practice Models? *13*
    Lois M. Stalling-Weldon, Cherona Hajewski, and Maria R. Shirey

    Learning From the Field: Consistency Between a Specialty's
    Recommendations for Advancing Professional Practice and a
    Nursing Theoretical Model *15*
    Susan Chasson and Jennifer Pierce-Weeks

2. The Importance of Professional Practice Models:
   Appreciating Significance *19*

    Learning From the Field: The Value of Professional
    Practice Models *32*
    Linda Q. Everett

3. Professionalism, Interprofessionalism, and Leadership:
   Commitment *35*

    Learning From the Field: Building the Case for Nursing
    Professional Capital *43*
    Sue Lasiter

PART II. FROM DESIGN TO ENCULTURATION

4. Components of Professional Practice Models: Design   *49*

    Learning From the Field: Building the Patient Care Delivery System
Based on the Professional Practice Model—A Journey of Synergistic
Development   *73*
Barbara Summers

5. Application of Professional Practice Models: Implementation   *79*

    Learning From the Field: Importance of the Chief Nurse Executive
During Implementation   *107*
Janet Fansler

    Learning From the Field: Innovative Implementation Calls   *109*
Polly Roush

6. Assessing the Success of Professional Practice Models:
Evaluation   *115*

    Learning From the Field: How Unit-Level Formative Data Improved
Implementation Progress   *143*
Joanne R. Duffy

    Learning From the Field: Communication of Outcomes Data Using
Graphical Displays   *145*
Eileen Caulfield

7. Refining the Professional Practice Model Within a Health System:
Adaptation   *153*

    Learning From the Field: How a Professional Practice
Model Together With a Spirit of Inquiry Led to a Practice
Adaptation   *168*
Martha Sleutel, Janet Larrimore, and Malika Qureshi

8. Translating a Professional Practice Model Into Everyday Practice:
Adoption   *173*

    Learning From the Field: Individual Adoption of the
Quality-Caring Model©   *185*
Shauna Bendix

9. Values and Behaviors Associated With Exemplary Professional Practice:
Enculturation   *189*

    Learning From the Field: How Our Professional Practice Model
Became a Magnet® Exemplar   *208*
Mary Teague, Debbie Manns, and Martha Sleutel

PART III. FROM APPLICATION TO IMPACT

10. Enduring Professional Practice Models: Sustainment   *215*

Learning From the Field: Professional Practice Model
Sustainability   *227*
Judy E. Davidson

11. Spreading Lessons Learned and Best Practices: Dissemination   *235*

Learning From the Field: An Interview With Two Vice Presidents
on "Scaling Up"   *252*
Alice Siehoff and Susan Okuno-Jones

12. Power of Professional Practice Models: Impact   *257*

Learning From the Field: Impact of a Living Professional Practice
Model on a Patient's Question—"How Long Would It Take
to Die?"   *269*
Pamela Duncan and Chantel Fusco

Afterword   273

Appendix A. Example: Values Clarification Workshop   277

Appendix B. Example: Implementation Booster Sessions   279

*Appendix C. Example: Organizational Assessment of Professional Practice
Model Integration   281*

Index   287

Contributors

Shauna Bendix, RN, BS, Novant Health, Prince William Medical Center, Manassas, Virginia

Eileen Caulfield, PhD, RN, NEA-BC, Director, Nursing Practice, Education & Research, Novant Health, Prince William Medical Center, Manassas, Virginia

Susan Chasson, MSN, JD, SANE-A, Statewide Sexual Assault Nurse Examiner Coordinator, Utah Coalition Against Sexual Assault, Provo, Utah

Judy E. Davidson, DNP, RN, FCCM, FAAN, Evidence-Based Practice/Research Nurse Liaison, University of California San Diego Health System, San Diego, California

Pamela Duncan, MSN, RN, CCRN, Manager, Nursing Professional Development, Moffitt Cancer Center, Tampa, Florida

Linda Q. Everett, PhD, RN, NEA-BC, FAAN, Former Executive Vice President, Chief Nurse Executive, Indiana University Health, Indianapolis, Indiana

Janet Fansler, DNP, RN, CNEP, Executive Vice President, Chief Nurse Executive, and Chief Operations Officer, Lakeland Regional Medical Center, Lakeland, Florida

Chantel Fusco, BSN, RN, Nurse Resident, Moffitt Cancer Center, Tampa, Florida

Cherona Hajewski, DNP, RN, NEA-BC, Vice President, Patient Care Services and Chief Nursing Officer, Deaconess Hospital, Evansville, Indiana

Janet Larrimore, BNS, RN, Patient Care Facilitator, Texas Health Resources, Denton Regional Hospital, Denton, Texas

Sue Lasiter, PhD, RN, Assistant Professor, Indiana University School of Nursing, Indianapolis, Indiana

Debbie Manns, MSN, RN, CPAN, Post-Anesthesia Care Unit, Texas Health Resources, Arlington Memorial Hospital, Arlington, Texas

Susan Okuno-Jones, DNP, MSN, MA, RNC, RN-BC, NEA-BC, Vice President, Nursing Practice and Innovation, Advocate Health Care, Downers Grove, Illinois

Jennifer Pierce-Weeks, RN, SANE-A, SANE-P, Education Director, International Association of Forensic Nurses, Elkridge, Maryland

Malika Qureshi, BSN, RN, Pediatric Staff Nurse, Texas Health Resources, Denton Regional Hospital, Denton, Texas

Polly Roush, MSN, RN, Senior Director, Novant Health, Prince William Medical Center, Manassas, Virginia

Maria R. Shirey, PhD, MBA, RN, NEA-BC, ANEF, FACHE, FAAN, Assistant Dean, Clinical and Global Partnerships; Professor, Department of Family, Community and Health Systems, School of Nursing, The University of Alabama at Birmingham, Birmingham, Alabama

Alice Siehoff, DNP, MS, RN-BC, NEA-BC, Vice President, Clinical Development, Advocate Health Care, Downers Grove, Illinois

Martha Sleutel, PhD, RN, CNS, Nurse Scientist, Texas Health Resources, Arlington Memorial Hospital, Arlington, Texas

Lois M. Stalling-Weldon, DNP, RN, CNS, Clinical Nurse Specialist, Deaconess Hospital, Evansville, Indiana

Barbara Summers, PhD, RN, NEA-BC, FAAN, Professor and Chair, Department of Nursing, Chief Nursing Officer, MD Anderson Cancer Center, Houston, Texas

Mary Teague, BSN, RN, CHPN, Nursing Supervisor, Oncology/Hospice/Outpatient Units, Texas Health Resources, Arlington Memorial Hospital, Arlington, Texas

Foreword

As a "seasoned" nurse executive, I frequently count my blessings, crediting the many nurse mentors, role models, and experiences I have interacted with for informing my administrative practice. As a nurse executive of a Magnet®-designated organization and the editor-in-chief of *The Journal of Nursing Administration*, I am often called upon to mentor nurses for leadership roles or to disseminate information through publications. This work, *Professional Practice Models: Successful Health Systems Integration*, by Dr. Joanne R. Duffy, should serve as a reference guide for nurse leaders, new nurse executives, and all faculty. Rarely has there been a comprehensive work of this magnitude produced to provide intense and practical direction for so many levels of practice.

As Dr. Duffy states in her text, we are undergoing rapid change in health care delivery. One stressor impacting the survival of nursing leadership and administrative practice is the impending number of experienced and highly successful nurse executives who are retiring or leaving their roles. This book by Dr. Duffy is a must-read for new nurse leaders following in our footsteps. It will enable them to increase their knowledge of the systems and processes required to implement, sustain, and measure professional nursing practice while providing a strategic framework to guide strategies for patient care.

Many experienced nurse executives have programs and initiatives in place to enhance the adoption of evidence in practice; however, few can show sustainable outcomes and consistent implementation of these practices by clinical nurses and leaders. This book will help provide practical guidance to support an understanding of roles in the implementation of professional nursing practice and the resultant application of evidence at all levels, including for students, clinical nurses, researchers, faculty, and nurse leaders. By sharing this book with others, nurse leaders can move through an organized planning process to develop structures for their own nursing organizations.

As an editor, I frequently receive manuscripts from writing teams presenting examples of innovations and improvements in care delivery. Few organizations have developed comprehensive practice frameworks to move beyond episodic projects toward sustainable change. Dr. Duffy provides a step-by-step guide for a more thoughtful approach through her practical implementation advice, case studies, and suggestions for systematic measurement and dissemination.

As an international researcher focused on the implementation of caring in practice, Dr. Duffy interweaves this component into the book. Caring practices and principles have been adopted by many organizations as a cornerstone of their nursing philosophy. Dr. Duffy provides a guide to take this well-known and proven theoretical principle and use it in understandable and easily demonstrable practice behaviors to support professional practice models.

Lastly, this comprehensive work supports our transition to new models of care, including population health. Nurse leaders are being challenged to assume new roles and develop new competencies. Through Dr. Duffy's work, the essentials of professional nursing practice will be developed, enhanced, measured, and preserved, contributing to new levels of wellness for our communities across the continuum.

Karen S. Hill, DNP, RN, NEA-BC, FACHE, FAAN
Editor-in-Chief
The Journal of Nursing Administration
Chief Operating Officer/Chief Nursing Officer
Baptist Health Lexington
Lexington, Kentucky

Foreword

The health care delivery system is undergoing extraordinary transformation shaped by changes in financing, access to services, availability of health professionals, and consumer demands. Nursing must be prepared to build on its professional practice model to generate innovative programs that enable nurses to practice efficiently and effectively. It is essential that members of the health profession work to improve the quality and safety of services that consumers receive. Professional practice models provide the framework for nurses to plan, deliver, and evaluate interventions that result in positive clinical and service outcomes. The multiple examples presented in this publication, *Professional Practice Models in Nursing: Successful Health System Integration,* are valuable resources for executives, nurse leaders, educators, and advance practice and staff nurses to create and deploy professional practice models to meet health system demands. The book is organized with powerful "Lessons Learned" stories for readers' consideration in their practice. Practice models that are person centered and evidence based are the basis for the delivery of excellent nursing care for all who trust us with their lives within and outside acute care settings.

Linda Burnes Bolton, DrPH, RN, FAAN
Vice President and Chief Nursing Officer
Cedars-Sinai Medical Center
Los Angeles, California
President, American Organization of
Nurse Executives, 2015–2016

Foreword

Health care is changing before our very eyes; in fact, we won't recognize it 10 years from now. The forces at play accelerating this transformation include moving from fee-for-service to value-based purchasing, the aging of the population, and the often unimaginable pace of technology development. Nurses, as the largest profession within health care, have an opportunity to be leaders in this transformation. One of the recommendations listed in the Institute of Medicine report *The Future of Nursing: Leading Change, Advancing Health* (2010) is to prepare and enable nurses to lead change. Harnessing the full potential of each and every nurse in the United States can improve the value of the entire health care system.

Practicing nursing at its full potential is best accomplished with a professional practice model fully integrated in places where nurses work. As of this writing, there are 423 Magnet®-designated facilities in the United States, and evidence continues to show that these health systems have lower mortality rates than their non-Magnet counterparts (Friese, Xia, Ghaferi, Birkmeyer, & Banerjee, 2015). An essential component of Magnet designation is having a robust, fully implemented professional practice model. *Fully implemented* is the key. The situation surrounding practice models is not unlike the famous strategic plan in which hours are spent crafting the words just right and then the plan lands in a file until it is time to review the plan's progress several years later. Professional practice models also face the same risk when a lot of time is spent selecting the tools and educating the nurses but little is done to hardwire the model into true everyday practice.

Dr. Joanne R. Duffy is an authority in developing practice models. Her Quality-Caring Model© has been successfully implemented in settings large and small. This text effectively creates a blueprint for how to make this process as meaningful as possible regardless of the model chosen or the type of organization considering the model. As an executive at Children's Mercy–Kansas City when it was receiving its first Magnet designation in 2003, I have seen firsthand the impact that can be made when these broad steps are followed.

One of the key points that is often missed and that Dr. Duffy clearly illustrates is the critical importance of evaluation. Historically, nurses and others focus a great deal on process measures. Although an important consideration, these measures mean little without strong evaluation of outcome measures. Process measures are important; however, the ultimate value of nurses practicing to their fullest potential is demonstrated through improved outcomes of care. This is an important means by which the value and contribution of nurses is better understood and viewed as more than just a component of the bed charge.

Dr. Duffy's blueprint is helpful whether you are a chief nursing officer (CNO), a Magnet or quality-improvement (QI) coordinator, an educator, or a student. The changes in health care will cause some organizations to make decisions that are reactionary and financially based. Nursing is always at risk in these situations because it represents a large proportion of labor expenses in a health system. A well-established professional practice model can help guide the organization generally, and nursing leadership specifically, to collaboratively make the best decisions possible while ensuring positive outcomes for patients and families.

An integrated and successful implementation of a professional practice model also ensures that important nursing values and how care is actually delivered are aligned between leaders and practicing nurses. If practicing nurses and nurse leaders make decisions together based on the professional practice model, this collaboration provides an opportunity for open discussion and creates a mutually beneficial and respectful relationship that is transparent and patient centered. Unfortunately, I often hear examples from around the country in which practicing nurses have inappropriate workloads and little support. This leads to disillusioned nurses who suffer from disengagement and ultimately moral distress and caregiver fatigue. A professional practice model can be the framework for productive dialogue that prevents these ill effects. In a time when there is a call for interprofessional teamwork in health care, it is imperative that we have our own profession in order.

Professional Practice Models in Nursing: Successful Health System Integration is an important text for those wanting to better understand this topic. The principles, rationale, best-practice examples, and reflective questions include crucial information needed to fully integrate professional practice models. The author delivers one of the most important works on this topic to date.

Karen Cox, PhD, RN, FACHE, FAAN
Executive Vice President/Co-Chief Operating Officer
Children's Mercy Hospitals and Clinics
Kansas City, Missouri
President-elect, American Academy of Nursing

REFERENCES

Friese, R. C., Xia, R., Ghaferi, A., Birkmeyer, J. D., & Banerjee, M. (2015). Hospitals in "Magnet"® program show better patient outcomes on mortality measure compared to non-"Magnet" hospitals. *Health Affairs, 34*(6), 986–992.

Institute of Medicine. (2010). *The future of nursing: Leading change, advancing health.* Retrieved from http://books.nap.edu/openbook.php?record_id=12956&page=R1

Preface

Central to the advancement of a health system is its workers, who today face many challenges, including less time with patients and families, burdensome regulations and increased documentation requirements, an aging and transcultural peer group, looming retirements, inadequate training and continuing development, and, at times, uninspiring leadership, all of which contribute to work-related stress. Professional nurses, the largest category within this group, face their own disciplinary issues of professional identity, entry into practice, delegation and accountability for care assigned to unlicensed personnel, integrating evidence-based practice into clinical workflow, and continuous change. As a result, nurses often find themselves practicing repetitive and often uninteresting work that is disconnected from its disciplinary source. And nurse leaders struggle to integrate large-scale change, oftentimes doing so imperfectly. Although the American Academy of Nursing's Magnet® program has enabled many health systems to distinguish themselves as exemplary in nursing practice by meeting several criteria intended to support nursing autonomy, empowerment, innovation, and high-quality patient care, there remains considerable controversy over the meaning of exemplary nursing practice and, in particular, how professional practice models as one source of evidence are successfully integrated into health systems.

As of this writing, over 423 health care organizations are currently designated as Magnet organizations (with many more on the "journey"). A key component of this recognition for excellence in nursing is exemplary professional practice as evidenced by a professional practice model that delineates the role of nursing, its relationships with others, how it is applied and continuously revised in everyday practice, by what means decisions about practice are made, how superior nursing practice is recognized and rewarded, and, most important, how nursing professional practice influences patient outcomes.

To meet requirements for Magnet designation, health care organizations expend valuable resources creating, implementing, and showcasing professional practice models, albeit using no coordinated or consistent approach, and often without attention to evaluation or dissemination of results. As a consequence, considerable variation in implementation and full enculturation exists, translation to the bedside may be lacking, limited empirical evidence of the value of professional practice models to patients or nurses has been revealed, and nurses and nurse leaders often become frustrated in their attempts to integrate such models throughout health systems.

The incongruity between the intent of professional practice models and the reality of health systems to integrate them into practice is notable and may be linked to worker dissatisfaction. Not only has professional practice model integration not been optimized, but improved outcomes as a result of their assimilation into nursing practice have not been adequately demonstrated, leaving the discipline without important evidence of the models' contribution.

Although most professional nurses and their leaders strive to practice in accord with professional values, many find themselves beleaguered with the challenging task of translating a multicomponent framework into long-standing hierarchical structures (aka compliance cultures) using traditional processes, particularly given the current realities of today's health care system. More specifically, in the midst of struggling to deliver high-value services, increase market share, and engage employees, many nurse leaders find themselves attending to elaborate performance improvement systems, expensive renovations, new regulations, and designer technology versus the practice of professional nursing. And registered nurses, who make up the largest of health professions and who spend the longest periods of time with patients and families, have a great need to practice from a disciplinary base, strengthen their accountability for quality patient outcomes, and find meaning in their work.

This book provides an overview of nursing professional practice models; their potential value to patients, nurses, and health systems; an orderly process of ensuring their translation into daily workflow; and the requisites for demonstrating their impact. The text highlights the contribution that exemplary professional nursing practice can make to patients, families, professional nurses, and the health care system, given a systematic and thorough approach to its integration. *Professional Practice Models in Nursing: Successful Health System Integration* builds on the professional literature, the author's experience integrating professional practice models, and emphasizes a systematic, evidence-based approach that takes advantage of nurses and nurse leaders working side by side in mutually beneficial relationships to promote optimistic and prosperous futures.

The intent of the book is to raise awareness of the significance of nursing professional practice models for improving the value of health services. Additionally, it is a resource for nurses and nursing leaders as they go about implementing such models, for students who are learning about nursing or health systems administration, and for educators who are teaching such content. Through the lenses of innovation theories, evaluation models, implementation and dissemination frameworks, and exploration of selected concepts such as individual adoption and organizational enculturation, the progression of professional practice model integration is presented. The importance of evaluation, sustainment, and generating impact is illuminated with multiple examples.

This author's knowledge about successful integration comes from a combination of the inclusion of her middle-range theory into many professional practice models throughout the country, successful national demonstration projects, her firsthand experience working with health systems as they implement and evaluate professional practice model integration, and her knowledge and practical application of theory and evaluation methods. Lessons from the field and reflective questioning, incorporated throughout the text, provoke important observations and useful insights that are beneficial for contemporary nurses and nurse leaders.

Part I focuses on the definition, value, and disciplinary need for professional practice models, and includes practical steps required in preparation for model integration. It is intended to provide a better understanding of professional practice models and to facilitate commitment to action. The next section is the mainstay of the text and, using various frameworks, discusses the processes of innovation and transformation that health systems experience as professional practice models are successfully integrated. It includes the design, implementation, evaluation, adaptation, adoption, and enculturation processes. The emphasis of Part II is eventual enculturation and it fulfills this purpose through repeated examples and exemplars, concentrating on the nurse–nurse leader relationship and associated strategies. The how-to's of values clarification, choosing a theoretical framework, specific implementation strategies, maintaining the momentum, and tipping points and milestones are addressed. It is important to note that evaluation and revision of professional practice model implementation, an often underrepresented aspect, is described in detail with attention to the author's personal experiences. Part III centers on sustaining the "transformed culture" and spreading professional practice models through specific communication mechanisms, and special relationships and practices. This part of the book concludes with a chapter on creating impact—influencing change beyond the doors of a single organization—adding value, and building an impressive future. Examples and other resources are presented in the appendices.

HOW TO USE THIS BOOK

The text is intended for use by nursing students, particularly graduate students and nursing scholars, as well as clinical nurses, nurse educators, nurse researchers, and those in nursing leadership positions at all levels. Magnet coordinators and health professionals in other disciplines may also find it helpful. Each chapter contains objectives, insets, a section called "Learning From the Field," key summary points, and reflective exercises designed to provoke thinking and application. As a whole, the text offers multiple examples and practice insights from diverse community and academic health centers, helping readers relate to the content. The appendices provide additional resources for those interested in implementation strategies and assessing the progression of professional practice model integration in their health systems.

Little has been done in terms of generating evidence for particular professional practice models and, in most health systems today, nurses still practice according to the biomedical paradigm amid the complexities of technology, multiple procedures, throughput, workflow, and supervisory roles. Although many health systems have embraced a more disciplinary perspective in their quest for nursing excellence, there remains considerable variation and, in some cases, utter confusion about the nature and full enculturation of professional practice models. In fact, many are confused about just what a professional practice model is and how it can enrich the practice of nursing as well as positively impact patients and the larger health system. A systematic approach to professional practice model integration fills a void in the literature by offering an established approach to implementation, suggesting methods for evaluation and revision and providing both practical lessons from the field and opportunities for reflection. This volume consolidates available information on the topic in one place, ultimately guiding nurses, nurse leaders/administrators, and educators in the process of translating professional practice models into clinical workflow, advancing nursing practice, and improving the quality of patient care.

Comprehensive integration of professional practice models offers possibilities for improving health outcomes, strengthening professional nursing practice, and providing exciting opportunities for ongoing research that will provide empirical evidence of their value. Especially during this period of transition in health systems, the challenge to nurses and nurse leaders at all levels is to ensure congruency between professional nursing values and professional practice. In doing so, they will preserve the timeless values that undergird nursing, deliver high-value services to patients and families, and provide meaningful work for practicing nurses.

Joanne R. Duffy

Acknowledgments

Thank you to all the smart, creative, and caring nurses—the most valuable health system resource—who have touched me in so many ways throughout the years. You know who you are, for we share many fond memories, amazing war stories, heartrending moments, and a common disciplinary connection. I watch in admiration those of you who are still "in the trenches" providing direct care to our most vulnerable; to others of you who are now retired but caring for grandchildren, parents, or "giving back" in some other way; to those who are instilling disciplinary values to our future graduates while pursuing important research questions; and to those inspiring nurse leaders who have challenged me in some way. Your professional contribution to patients, families, and society is profound, continuing to shape healthier lives. To you, I owe my deepest gratitude for providing me with a listening ear, the courage to persist, many laughs, and meaningful work that has made all the difference!

And to those nurses from all levels of health care who have voluntarily contributed to this book through "Learning From the Field" entries, you have enriched the text immensely. To all of you, your perspectives and wisdom provide the readership with valuable insights and lessons learned that would not otherwise be shared.

PART I

From Awareness to Commitment

Professional Practice Models: Raising Awareness

Professional practice models (PPMs), models of care, professional practice model components

By the end of this chapter, readers will be able to:

1. Summarize a professional practice model
2. Compare traditional and contemporary components of professional practice models (PPMs)
3. Distinguish between PPMs and patient care delivery systems (PCDSs)
4. Evaluate patient, nursing, and health system implications of PPMs

DEFINITION OF A PROFESSIONAL PRACTICE MODEL

Professional practice models (PPMs) are frameworks or systems that uphold and define the professional practice of nursing in an organization. Ideally, PPMs provide structure for nursing practice that is consistent with professional values, creates meaning for nurses, and offers benefits to patients and families. Such models help RNs feel connected to their own professional values, see the link between their own practice and the work of the institution, and showcase nursing's contribution to health care. More specifically, PPMs make visible the often invisible work of nursing. In doing so, RNs are often better able to focus on the priorities of their practice, set goals, improve their practice, and use the framework to guide research, thereby demonstrating the effect of their practice.

Hoffart and Woods (1996) first defined a PPM as a "system (structure, process, and values) that supports RN control over the delivery of nursing care and the environment in which care is delivered" (p. 354). The ultimate goal of a PPM is to improve the quality of patient care, but also to advance the practice of nursing by carefully delineating the roles and responsibilities of professional nurses and ensure their accountability for monitoring and evaluating performance. Thus, a PPM is a multicomponent system that serves as a guidepost for nurses and fosters the alignment of nursing practice with organizational priorities and professional values.

Often, a visual representation of a PPM is created and used by organizations to clarify the complexities of professional nursing practice. The resulting diagram depicts the various components of nurses' contributions and fits them together to reveal the entirety of nursing within a given institution.

COMPONENTS OF PROFESSIONAL PRACTICE MODELS

Traditionally, five coordinated components comprise PPMs, each building on the other and leading to exemplary professional practice that ultimately supports nursing autonomy, empowerment, innovation, and high-quality patient care (American Nurses Credentialing Center [ANCC], 2013). The five components include (a) the organizational mission and related nursing values or philosophy; (b) nursing professional roles, responsibilities, and relationships (typically derived from nursing theory); (c) a PCDS; (d) governance and decision making; and (e) a system of recognition/rewards.

Because the mission of an organization contains value statements and directs the energies of an organization, it is fitting that it provide the foundation for health systems' PPMs. For example, at the University of California San Diego (UCSD) Health System, the mission states: "to deliver outstanding patient care through commitment to the community, groundbreaking research, and inspired teaching" (UCSD Medical Center, 2014). As you might guess, ideas, such as stellar patient care, collaboration, commitment, research, and ongoing learning, could be gleaned from this mission. As it turns out, the resultant nursing philosophy statement is as depicted in Figure 1.1.

UC San Diego

HEALTH SYSTEM   <u>Philosophical Statements Supporting the Professional Practice Model</u>

These philosophical statements reflect upon the key values within the UC San Diego Health System professional practice model. We as professional nurses believe that caring relationships are at the core of our nursing practice. We care for our patients and their families, for our health care team members, for ourselves, and for each other as nurses. Our nursing practice is based on Joanne Duffy's Quality-Caring Model which explains that **feeling cared for** is essential to achieving exceptional outcomes. The goal is for all of us to "feel cared for" by embedding the following caring actions into our daily work of nursing.

Patient and Family
As professional nurses at UC San Diego Health System, we provide competent nursing care for all patients. Our practice is to be sensitive and caring while meeting the physical, emotional and spiritual needs of our patients and families. We recognize our patients' and families' unique experience including the uncertainty and vulnerabilities that accompany illness and suffering. As advocates for our patients we are present, genuine, responsive, sensitive, engaging, and assistive. Our **healing environment**, evidence based practice and **innovation** lead to stellar patient and family outcomes. Our goal is for each patient and family member to "feel cared for" during their experience at UC San Diego Health System. *WE CARE*.

Professional Nurses
As professional nurses we are autonomous and **accountable** for our nursing practice. Our practice is based on **research**, evidence and national standards. We are empowered to make decisions about our nursing practice through our **shared governance** model. Our clinical practice is caring, comprehensive, accurate and reliable. We pledge to engage in lifelong learning for our **professional development**. We take care of ourselves and develop caring relationships with other healthcare members so that we can develop authentic caring relationships with our patients and their families. As we develop caring relationships we feel cared for.

Health Care Team
We work collaboratively with all members of the health care team to provide **stellar outcomes** for our patients. We communicate openly and honestly in our advocacy for our patients. We conduct interdisciplinary rounds with the health care team and include patients and their families in the decision-making process about their care. We develop caring relationships with other members of the health care team so that they "feel cared for." Nursing leadership in clinical practice is evident at all levels and in all care environments within the organization. Nurses have a welcome voice at organizational meetings where decisions are made about care, practice, and the workplace. In all these ways, we, within the UC San Diego Health System, strive for nursing excellence.

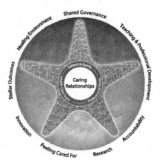

Our focus on developing caring relationships with patients, families, each other, and ourselves allows us to create an environment where feeling cared for is an everyday experience.

Figure 1.1 University of California at San Diego nursing philosophy statement (2014). Used with permission.

This mission and nursing philosophy advocate excellence through caring relationships, use of evidence, accountability, and teamwork that, one hopes, informs the subsequent roles, responsibilities, and relationships apparent in nursing practice. Using another example, at Indiana University Health, the mission reads: "Indiana University Health's mission is to improve the health of our patients and community through innovation and excellence in care, education, research and service," suggesting novel approaches to excellence, education, research, and service (Indiana University Health, 2014a). As it turns out, the nursing philosophy at the Bloomington, Indiana, hospital states: "nursing is a scientific discipline that takes a holistic approach to the diagnosis and treatment of potential and actual responses to illnesses. The goal of nursing is to lessen the effects of illness, promoting comfort and healing and assisting patients whether that is an optimum state of health or a dignified death" (Indiana University Health, 2014b). The mission and nursing values articulated in the philosophy statement suggest ongoing research and evidence—nursing is a scientific discipline—and holism, undergirding nursing's practice.

Nursing professional roles, responsibilities, and relationships comprise the second component of PPMs and are usually derived from nursing theory (but are not required). In fact, many organizations successfully design their own descriptions of nursing's roles, responsibilities, and relationships. Others prefer to adopt an existing theoretical model that fits with the articulated mission and nursing philosophy. In this component, how nurses practice, collaborate, communicate, and develop professionally is addressed. What professional nurses actually do when they provide care to patients (e.g., their day-to-day role, including what they are held responsible for), how they function alongside others to complete the work (relationships with the health care team), and how professional nurses grow and develop (e.g., continuing education, advancement systems, competencies) requires quite a bit of forethought and consensus building. The UCSD Health System described earlier uses the Quality-Caring Model© (Duffy, 2009, 2013) to define nursing practice that considers caring relationships at the core of nursing practice and specifically defines the role of the professional nurse as "to engage in caring relationships so that self and others feel cared for" (p. 38), in order to positively influence intermediate and terminal health outcomes. On the other hand, the Synergy Model (AACN, 2014) describes nursing practice at Indiana University Health. In this model, the goal of nursing is to "restore a patient to an optimal level of wellness as defined by the patient" and is accomplished when "the needs and characteristics of a patient, clinical unit or system are matched with a nurse's competencies" (AACN, 2014). This component of PPMs must "fit" with the mission and nursing philosophy and drive the PCDS. See Figure 1.2 for a consistency example.

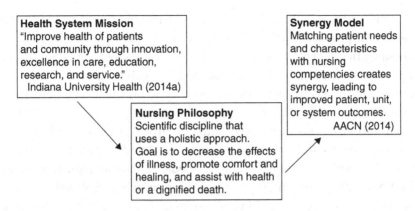

Figure 1.2 Consistency among organizational mission, nursing values, and nursing theory.

PCDSs detail broadly the various ways in which nursing work is coordinated and organized to meet patient care needs.

In essence, PCDSs include the wide range of practices and activities that occur in everyday settings where caregiving and care receiving are practiced (Lackman, 2012). PCDSs include work processes, communication patterns both within and outside the discipline (e.g., shift reporting, hand offs, interprofessional discourse), resources (e.g., staffing, assignments, staff mix), the context (e.g. the physical and cultural environment), and specific nursing interventions or practices derived from nursing theory that benefit patients and families (e.g., specific processes that nurses do with patients and families such as individualized education based on a health literacy assessment or a theory-derived intervention). In particular, PCDSs address professional nurses' scope of practice, continuity and transitions in care, accountability for clinical decision making, and outcomes. They also include how nurses are assigned to meet patient needs, what additional personnel are involved, who does what, and how patient care is recorded. Additionally, PCDSs describe the type and number of caregivers needed to carry out patient care. The work environment or the context of nursing practice is also considered. Organizational characteristics, such as leadership, support systems, and interprofessionalism, are components of the work environment along with the physical space. Finally, how nursing care is evaluated and modified is usually described in the PCDS.

Four traditional PCDSs—total patient care, functional nursing, team nursing, and primary nursing—have been used to operationalize the work of nursing (Tiedman & Lookinland, 2004). In total patient care, RNs assume complete care for patients. An example of this is private duty nursing or an intensive care unit or postanesthesia recovery room situation where an all-RN staff is employed. In a functional system of care, patient care needs were divided into tasks and distributed among a group of nurses and ancillary caregivers. For example, nurses, who were assigned to distribute medications for their shifts, administered all the medications to all patients on a unit or part of a unit. Team nursing used a system in which RNs led a team of unlicensed assistive personnel in the care of a group of patients, oftentimes defined by the geography of a unit (e.g., one wing). In the late 1970s and early 1980s, primary nursing, in which RNs assumed 24-hour accountability for patient care for a defined number of patients, emerged. In this PCDS, RNs used "associates," who could be other licensed professionals, or assistive personnel to guarantee that patient needs were met 24/7. However, the primary nurse assumed accountability for all care, including discharge planning and care that took place when he or she was off duty. Each of these PCDSs has benefits and challenges to nurses, patients, and health systems, although little systematic evidence has shown benefits of one system over another.

In more recent years, other PCDSs have emerged. For example, the Attending Nurse Model (Watson & Foster, 2003), which parallels the well-known Attending Physician Model; use of unlicensed assistive personnel in various nurse extender systems, such as the Partnered Model (Krapohl & Larson, 1996) or the Nonpartnered Clinical Model (Kenney, 2001); case management models (Girard, 1994); and, more recent, interprofessional disease management models for chronic care (Wagner, Davis, Schaefer, Von Korff, & Austin, 1999). In larger care delivery systems that go beyond nursing, such as accountable care organizations (ACOs) and patient-centered medical homes (PCMH), alternative models are developing. Regardless of the approach, PCDSs are one component of a PPM that is informed by the three preceding components: mission; nursing values; and nursing professional roles, responsibilities, and relationships.

How nursing is governed and decisions are made is the next component of a PPM. This component is closely related to the Magnet® criterion of structural empowerment and refers to those structures in a health system that support how decisions about nursing practice are made. It is linked most aptly to the concept of power, which implies authority, control, and the ability to influence or make decisions or to generate results. In nursing, it is only recently that power has been afforded to those who actually deliver care.

Shared governance, as coined by Cleland (1978) and later widely popularized by Porter-O'Grady (1992), is a system by which nurses control their practice as well as influence traditional administrative decisions. Shared governance programs typically are designed around committees that meet regularly and include staff nurses, educators, and managers who tackle issues such as practice, resources, quality and safety, education and development, research, and evidence-based practice (EBP). One approach is to organize several committees and have an overarching coordinating council that integrates decisions made by the individual committees. Another approach is to create a real Congress-type model in which representative nurses vote as a group on issues that directly impact their practice.

> Shared governance systems articulate how control over nursing practice is organized and facilitated in health systems and is guided by bylaws (or guidelines) that specify membership, terms of office, and decision-making processes and generate written proceedings.

Shared governance is predominantly about the *practice* of nursing, but often exercises some control over staff hiring, resource use, supplies and equipment, and other more administrative concerns. Although shared governance implies structure for decision making, it is the combined expertise, commitment, and accountability of the committee members that provide the "control" over practice. In fact, without these characteristics, few successes have been reported (Ballard, 2010). Fully mature shared governance systems provide the structure and processes necessary for nurse autonomy and empowerment.

Finally, recognition and rewards comprise the last component of a PPM and include how nurses are compensated, what types of recognition or awards are offered, and whether there is a career progression system that recognizes excellence at the bedside, typically called career ladders or career advancement systems. *Meaningful* recognition involves "acknowledging one's behaviors and the impact these actions have on others, ensuring the feedback is relevant to the recognized situation, and is equal to the person's contributions" (AACN, 2005, p. 189). Such recognition contributes to healthy work environments and has been associated with perceived organizational support (Kalisch, Lee, & Rochman, 2010), enhanced satisfaction and engagement (Carter & Tourangeau, 2012), and workgroup cohesion

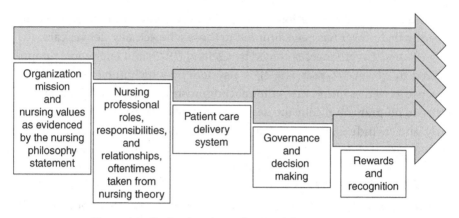

Figure 1.3 Professional practice model components.

(Cowden & Cummings, 2012). Although day-to-day personal recognition has been associated with enhanced self-esteem (Froman, 2010), organizational recognition in the form of annual honors, funding awards, clinical advancement systems, and public recognition of extraordinary nurses through professional associations or a system, such as the DAISY (diseases attacking the immune system) award (The DAISY Foundation, 2014), are examples of *meaningful* recognition. Obviously, how and what organizations choose to recognize and reward should be gleaned from the first four components of PPMs. The processes used to recognize and reward nurses strengthen the workforce by visibly celebrating the important work nurses do to improve the health of patients and families.

> Taken together, the five components of PPMs (Figure 1.3) provide the underpinnings for professional nursing practice in health systems, distinguishing its uniqueness and contributions. In particular, PPMs articulate the accountability nurses have to patients and families; uphold the specialized and ethical aspects of nursing; and provide interesting, meaningful work for professional nurses.

IMPLICATIONS OF PROFESSIONAL PRACTICE MODELS

Professional practice models have significant implications for patients and families, individual nurses, health systems, and the discipline of nursing. Anecdotal evidence has revealed improved outcomes in hospitals with well-defined PPMs and some evidence also exists for improved outcomes in those health systems designated as Magnet. As some have reported, nurses with higher educational levels or competencies delivered care that improved some patient outcomes (Kutney-Lee, Sloane, & Aiken, 2013); thus, nurse leaders must take seriously the nature of nursing professional practice at their organizations, analyze it often, and develop acceptable approaches for its enhancement.

> For patients and families, PPMs help RNs to focus on important aspects of practice that are theorized to positively impact patient outcomes. Emphasizing these components of nursing practice (over others) may contribute to improved safety, quality, and efficiency.

For individual nurses, PPMs provide the grounding for assessment, planning, implementation, evaluation, and documentation of nursing care. They also provide the basis for everyday work processes such as delegation, orientation and continuing education, decision making, assignments, and even how the environment or context is arranged. As members of a profession, individual nurses have an obligation to strengthen their practice and further their development. As such, actively applying PPMs to guide the nursing process and using them to inform clinical judgments and workflow decisions is crucial. Educators have a responsibility to ensure that professional nursing programs emphasize the components of PPMs so that graduates are prepared for the "real world" upon graduation. Related assignments, such as case studies, group projects, interviewing nurse leaders who use a PPM, and appraising the literature for evidence of PPMs, may enhance both undergraduate and graduate student learning.

PPMs have several implications for nursing leaders. First, recognizing that enculturating a particular model is a long-term process requiring top-level support, including adequate understanding of the model, visibility, high-quality relationships, accurate and timely communication, resources, and consistency of approach (walking the talk) is paramount. Second, depending on the level of leadership, ensuring that PPMs are implemented and evaluated systematically, consistency between model components is ensured, and the nursing workforce is empowered and enabled to assume accountability for "living" the chosen model are essential. Finally, attending to exemplary professional nursing practice can have a remarkable impact, provided it is authentic. Nurses and nurse leaders who are committed to a PPM exemplify its components, providing notable exemplars for others to imitate. In this way, health systems can embrace PPM as a way to increase organizational value by providing the means for full enculturation.

From a disciplinary perspective, PPMs have implications for professional roles and standards, the nature of interprofessional collaboration, documentation and information flow, performance evaluation, professional development and nursing curricula, and even funding priorities.

SUMMARY

The nature of a PPM, including its definition and component parts, was described. Components of various models were provided as examples and descriptions of PCDSs were presented. Implications for patients and families, individual nurses, health systems, and the discipline were offered.

REFLECTIVE APPLICATIONS

For Students

1. Discuss the components of traditional PPMs. Define each one. What contemporary elements could be considered as components of PPMs?
2. Analyze the PCDS at your organization. Is it documented? Does it flow from the organization's mission and is it articulated in the nursing value statement? Is it consistent with the professional roles, responsibilities, and relationships of professional nurses?
3. Explain how PPMs can inform the daily practice of nursing. Provide specific examples.

For Clinical Nurses

1. What new information did you learn in this chapter?
2. Analyze the PCDS at your organization. Is it documented? Does it flow from the organization's mission and is it articulated in the nursing value statement? Is it consistent with the professional roles, responsibilities, and relationships of professional nurses?
3. How were you prepared/unprepared for "professional" nursing practice during your educational program?
4. How can professional nurses use a PPM to modify nursing practice?
5. Do you participate in the governance system at your organization? Why or why not?

For Nurse Leaders

1. Does your organization have a defined PPM? Why or why not? If yes, what elements does it contain?
2. What components of a PPM give you the most pause? Why?

3. Create a plan for strengthening professional nursing practice at your organization. Share it with other leaders.
4. Think about the PCDS at your organization. Does it flow from the mission, nursing values, and articulation of nursing roles, responsibilities, and relationships? Why or why not? What do you need to do about this next?
5. How do you role-play exemplary professional nursing practice?
6. What "takeaways" can you describe from this chapter?

For Nurse Educators
1. Describe the courses in your curricula that discuss the PPMs. Critique and revise the content as appropriate.
2. Design a case study for baccalaureate students on the topic of shared governance. What is the scenario? What do you hope they learn?
3. What teaching strategies do you think would best guide graduate students in knowledge development related to PPMs?
4. Develop three learning objectives for a class on PPMs. How would you evaluate their attainment?

LEARNING FROM THE FIELD: WHAT ARE PROFESSIONAL PRACTICE MODELS?

For nurses practicing in *any* health care facility, the professional practice model (PPM) of nursing is a schematic description that clearly articulates how nursing is practiced in that respective health system. The nursing PPM is "the overarching conceptual framework for nurses, nursing care, and interprofessional patient care" (American Nurses Credentialing Center [ANCC], 2013, p. 41). The PPM "depicts how nurses practice, collaborate, communicate, and develop professionally to provide the highest-quality care for those served" (ANCC, 2013, p. 41). The PPM is an exemplar that demonstrates the manner in which nurses coordinate and provide patient-centered care, achieve best patient outcomes, and the manner in which nurses develop and perform professionally within their organization. Creating and embedding a PPM into daily nursing practice is a crucial requirement needed for nursing excellence.

Therefore, to facilitate achievement and sustainability of empirical outcomes within the organization it is essential to engage front-line nurses and nurse leaders in the design and dissemination of a customized PPM. Designing a tailored nursing PPM requires traditional, contemporary, and organizational components. Although traditional PPM elements include five broad subsystems (Hoffart & Woods, 1996), these elements might be too narrow in scope for today's complex health care environments, suggesting the need to incorporate a broadened definition of effective and efficient nursing practice (Miles & Vallish, 2010). Unique organizational factors also influence professional nursing practice; thus, the traditional PPM elements may coexist with more contemporary context-specific features.

Because a nursing PPM exists within a unique health system, designing it should take into account elements of the existing or desired organizational culture. Inclusive are hardwired structures, processes, and a culture supportive of a compassionate, evidence-based, and patient/family-centered care delivery model that achieves empirical outcomes. Health care delivery is also influenced by socioeconomic and technological factors that have significant implications for nursing roles and the manner in which patient care is delivered. Thus, contemporary PPM elements should reflect modern realities. For example, contemporary nursing practice and patient care management require care coordination and interprofessional collaboration across the continuum to reduce preventable errors and health care costs. Refining PPMs to reflect the ongoing transformation of patient care and health delivery systems from volume-focused to value-based systems is paramount. Finally, PPM elements that reflect expected nursing performance standards as well as recognition and reward systems should be included.

The value of a particular nursing PPM depends on whether the elements of the model contain well-established structures and processes that improve patient outcomes and reduce cost at both the microsystem and global level. The significance of an effective and well-designed PPM that drives down cost, maintains high patient satisfaction, and yields significant empirical outcomes demonstrates the contribution of nursing at the bedside. Likewise, an efficient approach to PPM enculturation substantiates justification of needed resources to sustain provision of high-quality patient care delivery.

Lois M. Stalling-Weldon
Cherona Hajewski
Maria R. Shirey

LEARNING FROM THE FIELD: CONSISTENCY BETWEEN
A SPECIALTY'S RECOMMENDATIONS FOR ADVANCING
PROFESSIONAL PRACTICE AND A NURSING
THEORETICAL MODEL

Since the 1970s, the care and evaluation of patients reporting sexual assault has increasingly become the responsibility of nurses. There are now more than 600 communities using sexual assault nurse examiners (SANEs) to provide this care. The development of a new specialty in nursing creates many challenges in terms of how to provide high-quality care. In 2006, the Office on Violence Against Women at the U.S. Department of Justice funded a project to look at the sustainability of SANE programs. Many of the recommendations made in the final report of this project support the use of theory, more specifically, the Quality-Caring Model (Duffy, 2009, 2013), as a foundation for providing exemplary care to patients who have experienced sexual assault. Recommendations from that project specifically identified changes in nursing practice that were consistent with key concepts of the Quality-Caring Model. See the following example recommendations:

1. SANE programs need to increase opportunities for staff self-caring by implementing peer debriefing to acknowledge the need for nurses to discuss their emotional reactions to providing this care.
2. Multidisciplinary teams should be implemented in order to better meet the needs of the patient, the SANE, and the community.
3. SANEs need to provide a more caring approach to survivors by "focusing on the healthcare of patients instead of focusing solely on forensic evidence collection" (Campbell & Patterson, 2014, p. 12).

    Each of these recommendations can be tied to a theoretical concept in the Quality-Caring Model and provide support for applying it as a foundation for practice. Additionally, the theoretical model "fits" with the SANE values of access to SANE nurses, fidelity to patients, responsibility to the public, respect for colleagues, and commitment to social justice. As new SANE programs are created and existing programs examine ways to strengthen and sustain their specialty practice, incorporation of the Quality-Caring Model could provide a powerful tool for guiding professional practice and ongoing development of this area of nursing.

Susan Chasson
Jennifer Pierce-Weeks

REFERENCES

American Association of Critical-Care Nurses (AACN). (2005). *AACN standards for establishing and sustaining healthy work environments: A journey to excellence.* Retrieved from http://ajcc.aacnjournals.org/content/14/3/187.full.pdf

American Association of Critical-Care Nurses (AACN). (2014). *The AACN synergy model for patient care.* Retrieved from http://www.aacn.org/wd/certifications/content/synmodel.pcms?menu=certification

American Nurses Credentialing Center (ANCC). (2013). *Magnet recognition program application manual.* Silver Spring, MD: Author.

Ballard, N. (2010). Factors associated with success and breakdown of shared governance. *Journal of Nursing Administration, 40*(10), 411–416.

Campbell, R., & Patterson, D. (2014). *SANE sustainability project evaluation: Final project report.* Enola, PA: National Sexual Violence Resource Center. Retrieved from http://www.nsvrc.org/sites/default/files/publications_nsvrc_reports_sane-sustainability-project-evaluation.pdf

Carter, M. R., & Tourangeau, A. E. (2012). Staying in nursing: What factors determine whether nurses intend to remain employed? *Journal of Advanced Nursing, 68*(7), 1589–1600.

Cleland, V. S. (1978). Shared governance in a professional model of collective bargaining. *Journal of Nursing Administration, 8*(5), 39–43.

Cowden, T. L., & Cummings, G. C. (2012). Nursing theory and concept development: A theoretical model of clinical nurses' intentions to stay in their current positions. *Journal of Advanced Nursing, 68*(7), 1646–1657.

Froman, L. (2010). Positive psychology in the workplace. *Journal of Adult Development, 17*(2), 59–69.

DAISY Foundation. (2014). *DAISY award.* Retrieved from http://daisyfoundation.org/daisy-award

Duffy, J. (2009). *Quality caring in nursing: Applying theory to clinical practice, education, and leadership.* New York, NY: Springer Publishing Company.

Duffy, J. (2013). *Quality caring in nursing and health systems: Implications for clinical practice, education, and leadership.* New York, NY: Springer Publishing Company.

Girard, D. (1994). The case management model of patient care delivery. *Association of Operating Room Nurses Journal, 60*(3), 403–405, 408–412, 415.

Hoffart, N., & Woods, C. Q. (1996). Elements of a professional practice model. *Journal of Professional Nursing, 12*(6), 354–364.

Indiana University Health. (2014a). *Mission, vision, and values.* Retrieved from http://iuhealth.org/about-iu-health/mission-vision-values/

Indiana University Health. (2014b). *Bloomington Hospital nursing philosophy.* Retrieved from http://iuhealth.org/bloomington/about/nursing-excellence/nursing-philosophy/

Kalisch, B. J., Lee, H., & Rochman, M. (2010). Nursing staff teamwork and job satisfaction. *Journal of Nursing Management, 18*(8), 938–947.

Kenney, P. A. (2001). Maintaining quality care during a nursing shortage using licensed practical nurses. *Acute Care Journal of Nursing Care Quality, 15*(4), 60–68.

Krapohl, G., & Larson, E. (1996). The impact of unlicensed assistive personnel on nursing care delivery. *Nursing Economic$, 14,* 99–122.

Kutney-Lee, A., Sloane, D. M., & Aiken, L. H. (2013). An increase in the number of nurses with baccalaureate degrees is linked to lower rates of postsurgery mortality. *Health Affairs, 32*(3), 579–586.

Lackman, V. D. (2012). Applying the ethics of care to your nursing practice. *Medsurg Nursing: Official Journal of the Academy of Medical-Surgical Nurses, 21*(2), 112–115.

Miles, K. S., & Vallish, R. (2010). Creating a personalized professional practice framework for nursing. *Nursing Economic$, 28*(3), 171–189.

Porter-O'Grady, T. (1992). *Implementing shared governance: Creating a professional organization.* New York, NY: Mosby.

Tiedman, M. E., & Lookinland, S. (2004). Traditional models of care delivery: What have we learned? *Journal of Nursing Administration, 34*(6), 291–297.

University of California at San Diego Medical Center. (2014). *Who we are.* Retrieved from http://health.ucsd.edu/about/who-we-are/Pages/mission.aspx

Wagner, E. H., Davis, C., Schaefer, J., Von Korff, M., & Austin, B. (1999). A survey of leading chronic disease management programs: Are they consistent with the literature? *Managed Care Quarterly, 7*(3), 56–66.

Watson, J., & Foster, R. (2003). The attending nurse caring model: Integrating theory, Evidence and advanced caring–healing therapeutics for transforming professional practice. *Journal of Clinical Nursing, 12,* 360–365.

CHAPTER 2

The Importance of Professional Practice Models: Appreciating Significance

KEY WORDS

Professional nursing practice, health system value, professional practice model (PPM) integration

OBJECTIVES

By the end of this chapter, the reader will be able to:

1. Describe the current context of professional nursing practice
2. Articulate how professional practice models (PPMs) contribute to health system value
3. Evaluate the preparatory steps for PPM integration

REALITIES OF PROFESSIONAL NURSING PRACTICE

RNs are practicing today in complex workplaces where financial pressures, regulation, advanced technology, looming retirements, globalism, acutely ill patients with never-ending needs, and multigenerational differences are commonplace, creating both demanding challenges and emerging opportunities. Difficulties, such as decreased resource allocation, overemphasis on routine tasks and documentation, employee disagreements, lack of support from ancillary services, compassion fatigue, and, most disheartening, uninteresting work, leave professional nurses frustrated and oftentimes yearning for alternative employment. Compounding this are the myriad organizational changes that leaders are demanding, many times without adequate evidence of their benefit.

To better understand the increasingly complex context of professional nursing practice, attention to the characteristics of individual nurses (education, credentials, unique life experiences, demographics), the characteristics of patients and families (acuity, age, life experiences, comorbidities), and the context (type of organization and its culture, how nursing is expressed and upheld, available resources, leadership, the nature of inquiry and creativity fostered, and relationships among the health care team) is warranted. These factors greatly influence professional nursing work, including its effectiveness in influencing positive patient outcomes. Although some of these factors are not under the direct control of nursing (e.g., patient characteristics), individual characteristics of nurses and how nursing is expressed and upheld in an organization are usually the purview of nursing.

Typically, some *individual* nursing characteristics become known during the hiring process, provided the process is thorough and can distinguish candidates who display professional behaviors, are nurturing, value lifelong learning, practice accountability, and can work together in teams from those who do not exhibit such characteristics. Once on board, individuals who tend to be more flexible, handle feedback positively, maintain their expertise, can regulate their emotions, are self-aware, and who cultivate relationships tend to perform better and are more engaged (Fujino, Tanaka, Yonemitsu, & Kawamoto, 2014; Schutte & Loi, 2014); these individuals exhibit high emotional intelligence (Goleman & Sutherland, 1996). These emotional characteristics can be influenced through ongoing continuing education, effective mentoring, specific professional development programs, and work experience; in essence, individual nurse characteristics can be molded by the context in which the nurse works (Goleman, Boyatzis, & McKee, 2013).

The expression of nursing professional practice in an *organization,* however, reflects how nursing is considered, conveyed, and claimed in an organization.

If nursing is considered a "profession" and its major concepts and scope are made explicit, the resultant practice will likely manifest specific values, activities, and interactions that reveal the full extent of nursing knowledge and skills.

For example, nurses who understand what concepts define their practice and who know the range of activities and interactions expected are more likely to adhere to those notions and perform accordingly. An example of this is demonstrated in a health system that distinguishes the use of the nursing process to provide *holistic* care that effectively meets patient and family needs, ensures that direct care nurses are engaged in practice improvement by participating in performance improvement or research councils, and enables interprofessional interactions characterized by inquiring, collaborative relationships. Such practice fosters creative patient-centered solutions. Typical performance in such a health system would be demonstrated by nursing actions, such as problem solving, analyzing, monitoring, teaching, counseling, decision making, improving, and relating, whereas fragmented, mechanistic-type work is likely minimized. When the major concepts and range of activities that comprise nursing are carefully considered, higher level professional knowledge and skills, for which nurses have been educated, may be better manifested.

These actions are *conveyed* to a health system through verbal and written statements, such as philosophies, clinical and system-wide policies, and marketing materials, as well as processes such as nursing representation on system-wide committees.

Conveying the scope and concepts that ground nursing practice in an organization implies written, face-to-face, formal, informal, electronic, group and individual communication and dissemination mechanisms that allow for questioning and feedback to ensure adequate appreciation of the role.

How a health system organization *claims* nursing professional practice is made visible through its hiring practices, performance expectations, professional development programs, and advancement criteria. Such processes, when infused with articulated nursing concepts and the full range of activities that professional nurses are educated for, tend to be reinforcing. Professional nursing practice that manifests in this manner is advocated for, defended, and rewarded, upholding the *professionalism* associated with nursing work. Although the context of nursing work is complex and dynamic, how it is expressed and upheld in an organization is an opportunity to create the energy for professional, interesting, and meaningful work (see Table 2.1 for a summary of these processes).

Table 2.1 Organizational Expression of Nursing Practice

Nursing Practice	Health System Processes	Resulting Performance
Considered	Nursing is thought about as a professional discipline (i.e., knowledgeable, competent, adheres to code of conduct and national standards, accountable)	Nursing activities and interactions exhibit the full extent of nursing knowledge, skills, and values
Conveyed	Verbal and written materials concerning nursing reflect its professional nature	Organization-wide appreciation of the professional practice of nursing
Claimed	Talent acquisition, performance expectations, and advancement criteria reflect professional ideals	Professional nursing practice is defended, advocated for, and upheld at all levels of the organization

THE VALUE OF PROFESSIONAL PRACTICE MODELS

Value connotes worth or merit of something (in this case a professional practice model [PPM]) and may also be associated with significance.

Professional practice models demonstrate nursing's contribution and project nursing's identity in an organization. As such, they hold value to patients, nurses, the discipline, and the organization.

Patients and families directly benefit from receiving care by nurses who practice under a PPM. More specifically, they can expect more commitment to professional values, accountability, ongoing competence, continuity, nurse input and collaboration on the interprofessional team (advocating for them), and creativity. Such behaviors translate into more robust decision making through increased reliance on evidence; caring for the "whole person"; individualized and participatory activities; new ideas solicited and welcomed; and full application of nursing's values, knowledge, and skills. Although little is known about whether PPMs actually improve patient outcomes (because few have studied this), it is rather intuitive that nurses who practice to their full extent would be a driving force in the attainment of health outcomes.

For nurses, a professional practice model depicts the major values and beliefs about nursing, identifies the parameters of nursing practice, including its responsibilities and authority for patient care, explicitly describes the systems for how nursing work is operationalized, and acknowledges expert practice.

PPMs offer nurses a way to appreciate their role expectations; facilitate a common language that is useful for communication; enable connections with patients, families, and others on the health care team; accelerate documentation; frame nursing interventions; and improve their practice. In essence, PPMs attend to the "voice of the nurse," empowering the nurse to advocate for patients and families, fulfill societal expectations, creatively innovate, and advance.

> Professional practice models support health systems by translating nursing concepts to the bedside, specifying the standards for nursing practice, enhancing communication, and reducing practice variation.

Although some practice variation may be beneficial, too much reduces effectiveness and efficiency. Take, for example, the routine of handwashing. In one Australian study using 30 nurses, the level of variation among and between nurses' reported practices and local policies was widespread *and* it extended across all aspects of handwashing practices—duration and extent of handwashing, type of solution, and drying method used (Morritt et al., 2006). It was proposed that nurses made their own risk assessments based on the proximity of the procedure to the patient. Despite the fact that hand-hygiene compliance has been continually taught and reinforced among health care providers and is linked to reduced hospital acquired infections and resultant costs, compliance with hand-hygiene guidelines has remained low (Larson, 2013; Sahay, Panja, Ray, & Rao, 2010). Thus, practice variation in this case may negatively impact patient and cost outcomes.

Contrarily, carefully establishing what nursing is and how it is operationalized in an organization may improve patient outcomes (e.g., safety, clinical outcomes, and the patient experience of care) and reduce costs (length of stay, supplies, and procedures). Additionally, because nursing practice is aligned with professional values, more satisfied and engaged employees may result, adding value to both patients' and health systems' portfolios. Nursing leaders and hospital administrators, who facilitate resources and provide the means for integration, can embrace PPMs as a way to increase organizational value.

From a disciplinary perspective, PPMs add value by providing clarity in terms of core competencies and role accountability (e.g., delineate differences and similarities among professional, technical, and assistive roles), may improve transfer of information and collaboration within clinical

teams, provide a method for evaluating performance, allow for benchmarking among similar organizations, and frame professional development
programs, including credentialing and self-regulation. Such transparency
informs nursing curricula, professional standards, practice improvement,
and even research funding priorities.

Based on the obvious value of PPMs to patients, nurses, health systems, and the discipline, it is reasonable to assert and pursue their integration as nursing responds to the current challenges in health care. Through
PPMs, an organization's values and mission are made explicit, shaping
resultant policies, including the compensation and advancement structure, resource use, the type and quality of services it offers, and ultimately
the bottom line! For health care systems, that bottom line is improved
patient outcomes, satisfied, engaged employees, and reasonable expenses.
Committing to a PPM, however, requires an understanding of the process,
including appropriate preliminary work, to satisfy the conditions for successful integration.

THE PROCESS OF PROFESSIONAL PRACTICE
MODEL INTEGRATION

Just as the management of patients and families is moving toward a coordinated continuum of care, nursing is shifting its thinking from separated,
geographic settings and task-oriented procedural functions to interde-
pendent, coordinated professionals working together over time to meet
unique, yet ultimately common, goals. Integration has been defined as
"the collaboration and linkages between and across organizational functions as well as organizational partners, including customers and suppliers" (Teixeira, Koufteros, & Peng, 2012, p. 73). This definition implies a rich
network of collaboration and information sharing among individuals and
departments, increasing transparency and feedback and the likelihood of
mutual problem solving. It also connotes better performance in terms of
quality and innovation. Successful internal integration helps create unity
among employees and alignment with the organization's mission. External integration refers to the collaborative involvement of others, such as
academicians, other health systems, customers (patients and families), and
even vendors, where trust, commitment, and information sharing become
the norm.

Integration of PPMs establishes harmony among nurses, nurse leaders,
various departments, other health care providers, patients and families, and
the overall health system, provided it is successful.

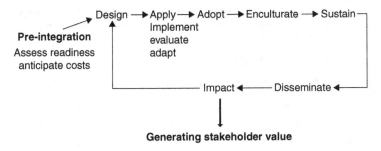

Figure 2.1 Phases of professional practice model integration.

The overall aim of integrating a professional practice model is to create a core platform of acceptable knowledge, behaviors, and values that define nursing practice and from which performance, specifically related to patient-centered health outcomes, can be optimized.

Professional practice models offer a shared mental image of the way nursing practice "could be" that drives interpretations and meanings, creates strong connections, and ultimately informs behaviors, shaping a coevolutionary culture (Korte & Chermack, 2007).

In practical terms, successful integration of professional practice models allows for common understandings, standards, work practices, and decision making to solve problems, make actionable improvements, and advance innovation, generating value for patients, nurses, and health systems.

Approaching integration in a systematic manner starting from assessing readiness to demonstrating stakeholder value is essential to its success.

In Figure 2.1, the integration process outlined in this text is depicted. It has been carefully thought out and applied in multiple health systems. The remainder of this chapter focuses on the preintegration phase and Chapters 4 through 9 will be devoted to the remaining phases.

PREINTEGRATION: PRACTICAL PREPARATORY STEPS

Nursing leaders are frequently faced with organizational change and its repercussions, especially those changes that involve modification of nursing practice or clinical workflow. The ability to adapt to such changes and alter the way nursing practice has been performed for decades requires a nimbleness that few health care organizations can quickly assemble. As a result, change

Table 2.2 Preparing for Professional Practice Model Integration

- Assess readiness

  Use internal and external evidence

- Conduct gap analysis (compare actual versus desired nursing practice)

- Anticipate costs

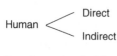

  Supplies and materials

  Opportunity

  Maintenance

is often incomplete, partially implemented, or abandoned altogether. In fact, in Senge's familiar *Dance of Change* (1999), the failure of most change initiatives to succeed at the "hoped-for" results, despite significant commitment of resources, is reported to be widespread. Kotter (2014), the well-known change expert, suggests that overcoming such setbacks requires fundamental shifts in thinking and doing—indicating that what is needed are dynamic, more flexible networks of individuals, who exhibit passion for innovation, are open to outside perspectives, appreciate human connections, and celebrate wins.

To be better prepared for the various nuances associated with integrating a PPM, nursing leaders should carefully consider how well they and their employees will accept and welcome the model (see Table 2.2). Such consideration generally consists of assessing evidence of readiness followed by a comprehensive strategy to alter existing practice.

Two forms of readiness evidence are especially helpful to better understand how well prepared an organization is to integrate a PPM. Foremost is the external evidence—that comes from the scientific literature and other organizations—augmented by the internal evidence generated from the integrating organization itself. Using both forms of readiness evidence creates comprehensive and compelling substantiation of an organization's preparedness for practice change.

Assessing Internal and External Evidence for Readiness to Commit

External Evidence

External evidence refers to the scientific literature and, in this case, to other organizations that have experience with components of the PPM in question.

Because PPMs are organization specific, only those components, such as the nursing theoretical base, specific patient care delivery systems, or shared governance approaches, may be represented in the literature. A review and appraisal of the literature pertinent to these components may provide evidence for a particular model component in terms of its possible inclusion, how easy it might be to implement and adopt, and how effective it was related to patient, nurse, and system outcomes. Another source of external evidence includes other health care organizations that use possible model components. By collecting stories and experiences from those organizations, one can elicit the quantity and types of organizations (e.g., community hospitals, academic medical centers, or free-standing clinics), patterns, and lessons learned. Finally, examining state nurse practice acts, standards of practice, and pertinent professional society documents provides additional evidence for consistency. Compiling such evidence provides a persuasive argument for selecting one model component over others.

Internal Evidence

Organizational readiness refers to members' change commitment and their efficacy in implementing organizational change (Weiner, Amick, & Lee, 2008). Or stated another way, organizational readiness refers to the degree that organizational members are psychologically and behaviorally prepared to integrate a new way of working. Transitioning to a PPM is smoother when organizational readiness is high and more problematic when the transition is viewed negatively or the organization just does not have the resources to successfully integrate it.

Because integration of a PPM into a health system is really about transforming a culture, evaluating whether or not a system stands prepared is paramount. Being prepared will support the process by ensuring that attitudes and suitable motivation exist in enough quantity to participate with the integration process and render it sustainable. The complexity of a PPM is critical for deciding whether or not it is appropriate for an organization to use. For example, some organizations design elaborate PPMs undergirded by complicated and language-sensitive theoretical concepts. Such models may inhibit full integration by creating unnecessary educational and resource requirements. Understanding this complexity is important to organizations in order to reduce the risk of wasting precious opportunities and resources, and/or harming existing nursing practice. It can also help to learn whether the leadership capacities of effective communication, facilitation, flexibility and responsiveness, evaluation, and staying the course are available in sufficient amounts to sustain the practice change.

Evaluating current conditions (existing structures, leadership, organizational culture, job descriptions), attitudes (political will, employee and leadership motivation, commitment), and resources (knowledge and skills, funding) of key stakeholders at all levels in an organization is important in order to understand whether the whole system or any of its component parts are ready. To do this, key stakeholders will need to know the scope of the PPM, including the requirements for personal, leadership, and contextual change. Lack of the right conditions, attitudes, or resources often creates barriers to optimum integration. Thus, understanding what and where these barriers are can provide valuable guidance for integration. For example, an identified barrier may have to be dealt with first, or the initiation of the model may have to be altered in order to "work around" an existing barrier that cannot be surmounted.

To assess organizational readiness for a PPM integration project, there are several questionnaires or tools that can be used to generate evidence of internal readiness (Holt et al., 2010). For example, the Magnet® gap analysis tool provides a short series of questions that are very specific to the program criteria and address some aspects of professional practice (American Nurses Association [ANA], 2014). Others are also available that assess readiness more broadly, such as the theory-based Organizational Readiness to Change Assessment (ORCA; Shea, Jacobs, Esserman, Bruce, & Weiner, 2014), which has two subscales: change commitment and change efficacy. Still other measures are available that speak to specific factors, such as employees' beliefs (Armenakis, Bernerth, Pitts, & Walker, 2007), or are unique to the health care context (Gustafson et al., 2003). Both employees and leaders alike should be the focus of such evaluations in order to obtain a more robust understanding of readiness to commit. Once this external and internal evidence is available, fully analyzed, and disseminated, organizational leaders will have a better notion of how well prepared they are for PPM integration.

Analyzing the Gaps in Nursing Practice

Actual performance (nursing practice) and desired performance (nursing practice guided by a PPM) of an organization represent a gap or a difference that provides additional data for leaders to use to evaluate the time and resources required to achieve full integration. Conducting such a gap analysis requires documentation followed by a leadership response.

Gap analysis usually starts with articulating the desired state. In this case, what would professional nursing practice look like after full integration of a PPM? For example, who would the practitioners be (characteristics, credentials), what would they be doing (job descriptions), when and where would they perform their work (scheduling and assignments), and how will that work be accomplished (workload, delegation patterns, interprofessional teams)? Next, it is necessary to document the current state with respect to each of the elements articulated in the desired state. This includes identifying who has the knowledge of the current state to answer such questions and determining how best to acquire this information. In some cases, there may be existing written records (e.g., staff schedules) or organization-wide documents (e.g., job descriptions) that can be used. In other cases, interviewing or assembling focus groups may elicit such information.

Once data is collected, quantifying it or collapsing it into categories of gaps, such as gaps in knowledge or gaps in resources, is crucial for clearly identifying the discrepancies between "what is" and "what should be." Although there is no *one* way of presenting discrepancies, it is important to display them in an organized manner. Finally, brainstorming together to develop strategies to "bridge the gap" or resolve discrepancies requires thoughtful dialog, creativity, and accountability, ultimately enabling the project's success. It is essential to assign the work to specific individuals with associated due dates in an effort to ensure accountability for the process.

Although assessing readiness evidence and conducting a nursing practice gap analysis are good ways to prepare for professional practice model integration, too much detail can overwhelm others, whereas too little detail will not provide enough information for strategy development. Thus, the goal is to include just the right amount of data to justify moving forward or pausing for a while to strengthen current conditions so successful integration can occur.

Using a shared, easily accessible electronic data file to identify key areas that are currently missing or inadequate, but that are needed for successful integration of practice change, represents an efficient way to prepare for successful integration.

Anticipating the Costs of Professional Practice Model Integration

Although adopting a PPM may offer a competitive advantage to health systems, it comes with a price. At present, cost pressures for health systems are escalating as decreased reimbursement rates, higher labor prices, lower

patient volume, electronic health record implementation, the unknown outlays associated with the Affordable Care Act, free care, and other expenses
intensify. In fact, the shift toward value-added care (health outcomes achieved
per dollar spent; Porter & Tiesberg, 2006) has substantially raised awareness
regarding the impact of nursing practice on costs. Thus, prior to integrating
a PPM, anticipating its costs is most beneficial.

How costs pertaining to PPM integration are most often delineated
(e.g., direct, indirect, opportunity, or maintenance costs) provides a logical starting point. Direct costs are those tangible expenses, such as the
cost of new equipment, salaries and benefits related to hiring additional
employees, engaging consultants, supplies and marketing materials, and
any required travel expenses, that are directly related to the PPM. Indirect
costs are those intangible outlays that affect the entire organization such
as charges for telephone and computer use, utilities, library resources,
administrative overhead, or rental equipment. Opportunity costs refer to
the costs of *not* implementing a PPM or how monies appropriated to PPM
integration could otherwise be spent. In other words, if nursing practice
remains stable in a certain health system while other close competitors
are incorporating a more professional way of practicing, how will the
estimated dollar value of that missed opportunity affect future revenue
streams? It could also mean what the organization could have done with
the available resources if they did not pursué the PPM. For example, if a
health system spent a large amount on PPM integration and then was not
able to offer wage increases for 2 years, how that decision affects employee
morale vis-à-vis local competitors might be a consideration. Finally, maintenance costs refer to the expenses associated with sustaining the PPM
after full integration.

Typically, PPM integration carries some elements of all four costs. For
example, direct costs may involve dedicating a salary portion of at least
one or, in many cases, several champions to facilitate model development
and integration, hiring a consultant to direct and inspire employees and
provide guidance on implementation and evaluation, costs for the development of an acceptable diagram that depicts the chosen model, employee
educational expenses, evaluation costs, and employee travel to other sites
and/or conferences. Indirect costs may include additional space for practice
model activities while the missed opportunity of *not* adopting a professional
practice must be analyzed in terms of an organization's standing among a
group of competitors. Ongoing costs, such as annual continuing education,

consultations, and evaluation, must also be considered. Thus, fully antici-pating the costs helps to prepare for better integration and sustainable results of PPMs.

SUMMARY

In this chapter, the realities of current nursing practice were described in light of ongoing change. How nursing practice is expressed in an organi-zation offers an exciting opportunity to depict how the practice of nursing contributes to the system while simultaneously showcasing how meaningful nursing work might be. The value of PPMs to nurses themselves, patients and families, the health system, and the discipline as a whole was discussed and made explicit through several examples. The process of integration, including the preintegration phase of assessing readiness and anticipating the costs, was explained.

REFLECTIVE APPLICATIONS

For Students

1. How do the realities of nursing practice discussed in this chapter compare to your notions of nursing?
2. What do you consider "interesting" nurse work?
3. Discuss whether nursing is a profession. Provide a rationale for your view.
4. What specific ways do you think a PPM adds value to patients and fami-lies? Why?
5. How would you go about gathering external data to support a PPM? How would you appraise it?
6. Develop a template useful for those completing a gap analysis.

For Clinical Nurses

1. What components of nursing work are "interesting" to you? Why? What suggestions do you have to provide RNs with more interesting work?
2. Analyze how your organization *expresses* nursing. Be specific—how is it considered, conveyed, and claimed? Does this affect nurses' views of their role? Does it affect patient care? Is it consistent with the professional roles, responsibilities, and relationships of professional nurses?
3. What sources of internal data are available at your organization to pre-pare for PPM integration? What could *you* do to help your organization prepare?

4. To prepare for PPM integration, what internal data are you currently aware of that might affect the model's success?

For Nurse Leaders

1. How do *you* provide interesting work for the nurses in your organization? What components are you involved in? How could you better advance an interesting work environment?
2. What components of PPM preparation worry you the most? Why?
3. Create a plan for gathering internal and external data, completing a gap analysis, and determining costs for PPM integration at your organization. Share it with other leaders.
4. Think about the internal characteristics at your organization. Are you ready for PPM integration? Why or why not? What can be done to increase readiness?
5. What "takeaways" from this chapter were most meaningful to you?

For Nurse Educators

1. Describe how the content in this chapter can be best translated to undergraduate and graduate students.
2. Using role modeling as a strategy, how could aspects of this chapter be demonstrated? What will you do? How will you ensure that cognitive, behavioral, and affective ways of learning are incorporated?
3. Develop a teaching strategy for helping graduate students understand the preparatory requirements of PPM integration.
4. How would you evaluate the chapter objective: "articulate how PPMs contribute to health system value"?

LEARNING FROM THE FIELD: THE VALUE OF PROFESSIONAL PRACTICE MODELS

Professional practice models (PPMs) are important because they provide the overarching conceptual framework for nurses, nursing care, and interprofessional patient care. They are quite literally the road map for excellence in care delivery—describing and depicting how nurses practice, collaborate, communicate, and develop professionally to provide the highest quality of care.

Demonstrated excellence in exemplary professional practice (the desired result of PPM integration) enables nurse autonomy, accountability, and authority, which positions nurses to advocate for patients. Indiana University Health believes that nursing is a profession, not an occupation, and members of the nursing team are clear on the difference. A robust PPM, supported by theory, centers the care delivery model that is grounded in a strong mission, vision, and a set of core values. Thus, a PPM supports nurses and team members as they deliver patient care.

In doing so, PPM support practice that is consistent with the tenets of the profession, including essential values such as altruism, equality, esthetics, freedom, human dignity, justice, and truth. Most important, PPM equally embody the rights of patients and the rights of nurses, enabling shared decision making at all levels, as well as ongoing professional development.

Evaluation of PPMs, both formally and informally, through established structures and processes, including shared leadership/governance mechanisms, provides evidence of system value and the basis for continuous improvement. Measurement elements should include patient satisfaction; evidence-based practice; RN professional development; RN reward and recognition; safe, timely, efficient, effective, and equitable patient-centered care; and RN satisfaction with decisional involvement, team relationships, resource adequacy, management, and workplace safety. Health systems and nurses desperately need these data to demonstrate their contribution to the highest quality of care.

Linda Q. Everett

REFERENCES

American Nurses Association (ANA). (2014). *Pathway to excellence®: Are you ready to apply?* Retrieved from http://www.nursecredentialing.org/Pathway/Pathway Pages/AssessmentGapAnalysis

Armenakis, A. A., Berneth, J. B., Pitts, J. P., & Walker, H. J. (2007). Organizational change recipient's scale. Development of an assessment instrument. *Journal of Applied Behavioral Science, 43*(4), 481–505.

Fujino, Y., Tanaka, M., Yonemitsu, Y., & Kawamoto, R. (2014). The relationship between characteristics of nursing performance and years of experience in nurses with high emotional intelligence. *International Journal of Nursing Practice.* Advance online publication. doi:10.1111/ijn.12311

Goleman, D., & Sutherland, S. (1996). Emotional intelligence—Why it can matter more than IQ. *Nature, 379*(6560), 34–35.

Goleman, D., Boyatzis, R., & McKee, A. (2013). *Primal leadership: Unleashing the power of emotional intelligence.* Boston, MA: Harvard Business School Publishing.

Gustafson, D. H., Steudel, F., Eichler, M., Adams, L., Bisognano, M., & Steudel, H. (2003). Developing and testing a model to predict outcomes of organizational change. *Health Services Research, 38*(2), 751–776.

Holt, D. T., Helfrich, C. D., Hall, C. G., & Weiner, B. J. (2010). Are you ready? How health professionals can comprehensively conceptualize readiness for change. *Journal of General Internal Medicine, 25*(Suppl 1), 50–55.

Kotter, J. (2014). *Accelerate*. Boston, MA: Harvard Business Review Press.

Korte, R., & Chermack, T. (2007). Changing organizational culture with scenario planning. *Futures, 39*(6), 645–656.

Larson, E. (2013). Monitoring hand hygiene: Meaningless, harmful, or helpful? *American Journal of Infection Control, 41*(5), S42–S45.

Morritt, M. L., Harrod, M. E., Crisp, J., Senner, A., Galway, R., Petty, S., . . . Donnellan, R. (2006). Handwashing practice and policy variability when caring for central venous catheters in pediatric intensive care. *Australian Journal of Critical Care, 19,* 15–21.

Porter, M. E., & Teisberg, E. O. (2006). *Redefining health care: Creating value-based competition on results*. Boston, MA: Harvard Business School Press.

Sahay, S., Panja, S., Ray, S., & Rao, B. K. (2010). Diurnal variation in hand hygiene compliance in a tertiary level multidisciplinary intensive care unit. *American Journal of Infection Control, 38*(7), 535–539.

Schutte, N. S., & Loi, N. M. (2014). Connections between emotional intelligence and workplace flourishing. *Personality and Individual Differences, 66,* 134–139.

Senge, P. M., Kleiner, A., Roberts, C., Ross, R., Roth. G., & Smith, B. (1999). *The dance of change*. New York, NY: Doubleday.

Shea, C. M., Jacobs, S. R., Esserman, D. A., Bruce, K., & Weiner, B. J. (2014). Organizational readiness for implementing change: A psychometric assessment of a new measure. *Implementation Science, 9,* 1–7. doi:10.1186/1748-5908-9-7

Teixeira, R., Koufteros, X. A., & Peng, X. D. (2012). Organizational structure, integration, and manufacturing performance: A conceptual model and propositions. *Journal of Operations and Supply Chain Management, 70*(1), 69–81.

CHAPTER 3

Professionalism, Interprofessionalism, and Leadership: Commitment

KEY WORDS

Professional practice, interprofessionalism, leadership, commitment

OBJECTIVES

By the end of this chapter, readers will be able to:

1. Differentiate between the terms *professional* and *being* professional
2. Apply the principles of interprofessionalism to the professional practice of nursing
3. Evaluate how the professional practice of leadership is tied to nursing professional practice models (PPMs)
4. Examine individual and leadership commitment to professional nursing practice

THE PROFESSIONAL PRACTICE OF NURSING

The practice of nursing is grounded by the American Nurses Association's (ANA) seminal documents: *Code of Ethics for Nurses With Interpretive Statements* (ANA, 2015), *Nursing: Scope and Standards of Practice* (ANA, 2010a), and *Nursing's Social Policy Statement* (ANA, 2010b) and further influenced by individual state nurse practice acts. These documents define nursing and nursing practice, describe how nursing practice fulfills society's mandate, present standards and competencies that influence the professional role of nursing, explain regulations that guide professional practice, and establish the ethical base for all nurses regardless of setting. Furthermore, the documents highlight the mutually beneficial relationship between society and the nursing profession (i.e., nursing's response to societal needs). Thus, individual professional nurses are responsible not only for their own behaviors but also to the needs of society or the community served. This "contract" that exists between nursing and society provides the authority to practice professional nursing.

In Nursing's *Social Policy Statement* (ANA, 2010b), theory application and use of research serve as the basis for nursing actions (or interventions) whose aims are to "protect, promote, and optimize health; to prevent illness and injury; to alleviate suffering; and to advocate for individuals, families, communities, and populations" (p. 10), leading to beneficial outcomes. Throughout these various documents, elements of accountability, including current licensure, delegation issues, continuous improvement, and leadership, are repeatedly presented. Understanding the content of these professional documents and "applying" them to everyday practice, however, are two different phenomena.

The shifting focus toward health system value (the Triple Aim; Institute for Healthcare Improvement [IHI], 2007) demands sophisticated application of professional nursing behaviors (e.g., *being* professional). *Being* professional relates to behaving in a manner that is expected of a professional (e.g., acting in accordance with the seminal documents previously described) as well as sustaining effective interactions, reliable behaviors, and autonomous commitment to continuous improvement (Wilkinson, Wade, & Knock, 2009).

In fact, *being* professional is hard work that some would say does not occur at a single point in time (e.g., during an educational program) but develops over time, maturing with knowledge, experience, and ongoing self-awareness.

Being professional encompasses specialized knowledge and skills, collaborative interpersonal approaches, responsiveness and revision of how one is perceived by others (e.g., physical appearance, stance, displays of human respect and compassion), ongoing improvement, and informed decision making. The term *professional comportment* has been used to describe this phenomenon and is defined as a "dignified manner or conduct" (Clicker & Shirey, 2013, p. 107) that is equal in importance to technical tasks.

Being professional is associated with knowledge of one's work (Drucker, 1994, 1999), which is important not only because it is tied to disciplinary ideals, but also because it adds value to those served as well as to the associated organizations. For example, how is a patient or family's experience shaped by a disheveled nurse with a passive stance versus a professional-looking nurse with an optimistic stance? Although anecdotal, many patients have reported to this author a remarkable difference in their willingness to disclose, adhere to the plan of care, or to trust health care providers based on their appearance and behavior alone. Thus, professional comportment must be developed and nurtured in health systems in order to successfully deliver care aligned with patients' preferences and values.

In the *Blueprint for 21st Century Nursing Ethics: Report of the National Nursing Summit* (Johns Hopkins University School of Nursing and the Berman Institute of Bioethics, 2014), nurse leaders acknowledged the ethical challenges that nurses face in everyday practice, but also committed to strengthen nursing's ethical foundation in order to meet the challenges facing health systems. In particular, they spoke to strengthening the context, clinical practice, education, research, and policy related to professional practice. Ideas, such as more intentional practice, accountability and personal responsibility, interdisciplinary efforts, acknowledging moral distress among nurses, the availability of adequate resources, and building on existing work—all features of professional practice models (PPMs)—were advocated.

Although most health professionals value their own disciplinary expertise and judgment, and display this through independent actions, working as a collaborative team member is also part of professional practice. It is only recently, however, that health professionals have embraced interprofessional practice to the extent that it is a crucial element of training programs. Fostering interprofessionalism through collegial actions that ultimately enhance patient outcomes is an expectation of *professional* nursing practice (Interprofessional Education Collaborative Expert Panel, 2011).

INTERPROFESSIONALISM

Interprofessional collaboration is crucial for meeting society's expectations for enhancing health. The World Health Organization (WHO) defines *interprofessional collaborative practice* as a process whereby multiple health workers from different professional backgrounds provide comprehensive services by working with patients, families, caregivers, and communities to deliver the highest quality of care across settings (WHO, 2010, p. 13). Interprofessional teamwork, on the other hand, refers to the quality of the team process and its goals, collaboration, mutual aims, and optimal communication (Thistlethwaite & Dallest, 2014). In other words, interprofessional teamwork is undergirded by the relational attributes of team members, the appreciation of others' goals, and mutual communication.

Several studies have demonstrated a link between interprofessional practice and improved patient outcomes (Reeves et al., 2009). Current delivery systems, however, frequently persist in organizing health professionals by discipline; staff work in separate clinical departments (Kline, Willness, & Ghali, 2008) that practice independently. Yet, the problems encountered by today's patients are often so great that well-intentioned health professionals cannot resolve them alone. For example, Mazzocco, Pettiti, and Fong (2009) found that patients whose surgical teams exhibited fewer teamwork behaviors were at a higher risk for death or complications, even after adjusting for patient risk.

Despite the renewed interest in the academic preparation for interprofessional practice, translation into health systems has been slow. Cashman notes, "absent structures and systems that support interprofessional *practice*, professionals run the risk of reverting to old, traditional modalities of parallel practice" (Cashman, Reidy, Cody, & Lemay, 2004, p. 184). Health professionals increasingly indicate the need to collaborate but changing long-established systems has been challenging.

Carefully insisting on the inclusion of interprofessionalism in PPMs is an ethical responsibility. Building relationships through role modeling interprofessionalism and empowering others to develop flexible and effective relationships that add value (e.g., enhance patient outcomes) contributes to interprofessionalism. Helping others to identify aspects of practice that require collaboration, to accept multiple perspectives, and to continually monitor and improve practice fosters the overall goal of "what's best for the patient," an ideal of all health professionals.

LEADING A PROFESSION

The Institute of Medicine's (IOM) report *The Future of Nursing* (IOM, 2010) advocated for nurses to take on greater roles in leading change to advance health care in America. This report called for leadership at all levels of nursing, and personal accountability for ongoing professional development, including interprofessional collaboration and coordination. More specific, the report called for transformative leadership that advances nursing's role as a full partner. Leading in this context calls for a more actionable approach that considers patient welfare as primary, and its continued improvement over time, essential. Although all nurses are considered leaders, some have organizational responsibility for leading groups of nurses in the delivery of patient-centered

> Leadership is a practice in its own right that complements clinical practice; it enjoys an evidence base and an associated body of knowledge.

care. Through repeated evidence-based work experiences, acquisition of new knowledge, and ongoing reflection, leadership proficiency evolves, supporting the hard work of health professionals in meeting society's needs for health and wellness. As such, leadership is a lifelong process of learning, performing, pondering, and performing again.

> As leaders of a profession, nurses are called to consider the patient (and by extension, the family) as their first priority and rehearse (over and over again) the practice they have been prepared to advance.

Those who formally lead the profession (such as those with administrative titles) must remember that they are "guiding a practice whose first responsibility is to patients and families, that bears responsibility for providing competent, high-quality services, and that is uniquely qualified to advance relationships that improve the human experience" (Duffy, 2013, p. 170). Thus, nurse leaders are in a unique position to facilitate professionalism by stewarding the integration of PPMs. Placing the patient and family at the center of professional practice and using their input in the choice, implementation, evaluation, revision, and adoption of PPMs supports the IOM definition of transformational leadership. Ensuring coordinated teams of professionals, who work together to achieve specific patient-centered outcomes in an efficient manner, facilitates nursing's role as a full partner.

COMMITTING TO PROFESSIONAL PRACTICE

Professional practice models empower professional nurses by providing the foundation and infrastructure to deliver high-quality patient care. Yet, dedicating time and resources to PPM integration requires steadfastness over time, especially during stressful periods, along with continued focus on the ultimate goal(s). In essence, commitment is the glue that ensures successful integration.

Commitment is a human phenomenon that helps us organize our behaviors. Whether it is visually observed or not, commitment connotes action of some sort and usually is tied to some future occurrence or outcome. Commitment in the context of PPM integration creates not only possibilities but expectations for others. Thus, without a determination about what is committed, others may not follow or share in the expectations.

Integrating PPMs in an established organization with traditional ways of practice is a long-term investment that carries upsides and downsides. For example, although initial enthusiasm might be high, as particular roles or responsibilities are eventually altered, individuals often lose interest.

To sustain the initial momentum, a different disposition is required— one that is less hesitant or cautious in favor of one that is more convincing or definitive. Such a stance is best held at the local (or unit) level where individual nurses who are passionate about the PPM work side by side with other nurses and can help them see the possibilities for a different, more professional practice. These nurse champions are enthusiastic, intelligent, and present opinions that others listen to. Of course, although such individuals can initiate momentum, long-term commitment is necessary, requiring an enduring presence to sustain new behaviors. Identifying and nurturing unit-level champions are key to maintaining commitment. The following exemplar represents one direct care nurse's evolving commitment to a professional practice model:

> As a BSN-prepared nurse, I learned a long time ago to be careful about trying new things. Once I became aware of our hospital's professional practice model, I was intrigued with the idea of practicing in a way that is true to my heart, but wary of how it might change my daily routine. After all, it had taken me a little over 18 months to become comfortable with the unit. But after I learned about the professional practice model, designed by the practice council, it didn't take much convincing for me to see how it might change practice for the better. Little by little I got involved in it by first getting educated on it, and then, following the lead of the unit charge nurse, helping with goals for implementation, redesign of the care delivery system, and eventually assisting with evaluation. More specifically, I provided input into the staffing mix, interprofessional rounds, and helped with communication. I educated the unit unlicensed assistive personnel in the revised nursing role, assuring them of their continued value to the team. This experience has reaffirmed for me that stepping out of one's comfort zone has many benefits, for me, my co-workers, and patients. I can't believe all I have learned. (Personal communication, September 23, 2015)

This exemplar shows the value of committed unit champions who, after identification and with a little encouragement, will help expedite integration by promoting the model at the unit level.

Finally, although unit champions are crucial to sustained commitment, those in formal leadership roles have the responsibility to psychologically align with the PPM (Herold & Fedor, 2008) and maintain a positive attitude toward the future when nursing practice will be more professionally based.

> Understanding and embracing the chosen model, demonstrating a certainty of what is not yet visible, the willingness to repeatedly share its benefits to others (including other health professionals and administrators), and using multiple methods in various formats to communicate it throughout the system are commitment behaviors that allow for successful integration.

SUMMARY

In this chapter, the meaning of professional practice is presented in light of grounding ANA documents and state nurse practice acts. Furthermore, the phenomenon of *being* professional with its intended accountability for effective interactions, continuous improvement, awareness of self, and use of evidence in decision making was reviewed. The term *professional comportment* was defined, whereas interprofessionalism and its link to PPMs was described. Finally, leadership practice and commitment as they relate to successful integration of PPMs were explained.

REFLECTIVE APPLICATIONS

For Students

1. Review *Nursing's Social Policy Statement*. How does this document help you understand your duty to society?
2. Think about the nurses you know or those you have seen in clinical courses. Are they *being* professional? What behaviors lead you to describe them this way?
3. Discuss the difference between professional practice and *being* professional.
4. How do you think others perceive you? Why is this important in patient care?
5. Explain your responsibility for collaborative practice. How would you evaluate your interprofessional performance?
6. Develop a list of behaviors you would like nurses to display that demonstrated commitment to professional practice.

For Clinical Nurses

1. What components of your everyday work are based in the ANA documents on professional practice?
2. Analyze how your peer group conveys *being* professional. Be specific— what does *being* professional look like? Do you think such behavior affects nurses' views of their role? Does it affect patient care? Why?
3. What does your stance say about you as a professional? How about your appearance?
4. To prepare for PPM integration, how will you facilitate nurses' commitment to the model?
5. What behaviors do you practice interprofessionally? How could interprofessionalism be advanced on your unit?

For Nurse Leaders

1. How are the founding ANA booklets and the state nurse practice act conveyed throughout your health system? How could you better advance nurses' understanding of these documents?
2. How do *you* convey *being* professional to those you supervise?
3. How is your leadership practice based on evidence? When was the last time you used current evidence to make a leadership decision? What was it? How did the evidence inform your decision?
4. Do patients and family members regularly contribute input to improving nursing practice? Why or why not? How could you facilitate their feedback?
5. How do you ensure that collaborative interprofessional practice is occurring in your health system? How is it evaluated and improved?
6. Are you committed to PPM integration? What leads you to answer this way?
7. Think about the characteristics of direct care nurses on your unit(s). Can you identify any early adopters? What about the early majority? Are you ready for PPM integration? Why or why not? What can be done to increase readiness?

For Nurse Educators

1. Describe how the content in this chapter can be best translated to undergraduate and graduate students?
2. What takeaways from this chapter have the most implications for education?
3. Are the ANA documents listed in this chapter used in your curriculum? Why or why not? What about the state nurse practice act?

4. How do you ensure that *being* professional is learned and incorporated into clinical practice?
5. What teaching strategies might best help undergraduate students understand the content of this chapter? Why?
6. How is interprofessionalism taught in your program? What could you do to enhance collaborative practice? Do you have any recommendations for fostering interprofessionalism during clinical courses?

LEARNING FROM THE FIELD: BUILDING THE CASE FOR NURSING PROFESSIONAL CAPITAL

After interviewing intensive care survivors for my dissertation research, I was buried in reams of qualitative data that represented the insight shared by patients about their perceptions of feeling safe in intensive care. Their narratives were mainly about nurses; what nurses knew, how nurses carried out their work, words nurses offered as encouragement, and how nurses could be counted on to come quickly when help was needed. It occurred to me that these patients were describing a concept that I call professional capital and were using facets of this concept to describe their nurses. Let me explain my reasoning.

Consistent with the definition of *professional*, nurses have a specialized body of knowledge that is learned through the study of nursing science (Merton, 1960). Through study, coupled with experience, nurses come to know their work and how to determine when it is effective and meaningful (Schinkel & Noordegraaf, 2011). Nurses place patient needs over personal and professional gain and demonstrate unrelenting ethical and moral commitment to patients by influencing public health and social welfare (Tarlier, 2004). These actions, along with relationships that are formed between patients and nurses, are noticed and valued by patients (DeFrino, 2009; Fletcher, Berg, Simmermann, White, & Behrens, 2007).

The term *capital* was first used in the 1800s by economists in reference to monetary and material possessions (Casey, 2008). Since then, concepts, such as *human, intellectual* (Covell, 2008), *symbolic* (Bourdieu, 1984, 1986), as well as *social* (Boix & Posner, 1998) have been added as prefix modifiers and used to describe people such that *human capital* refers to a person's knowledge, experience, and expertise. *Intellectual capital* is knowledge contributed by people within an organization, which becomes evident through better quality and better outcomes. Because nurses offer considerable human and intellectual capital, they are an indispensable part of the survival and advancement of health care organizations that seek to provide high-quality, patient-centered care. As patients recognize that an institution legitimately values and delivers quality care, the institution obtains symbolic capital. Additionally, social capital, the joint cooperation (and the joint responsibility) of all professionals within an institution who are focused on achieving common goals, is noticed and valued by patients.

Thus, the amalgamation of definitions plus quantitative polls and qualitative data serves as evidence that supports the case that nurses have demonstrated and possess professional capital in the following ways:

- Quantitative evidence has consistently shown public recognition of nurses as honest, ethical (Gallup, 2013), and trustworthy (ANA, 2013).
- Qualitative research findings have provided evidence that patients view nurses as knowledgeable and accessible and that positive patient–nurse relationships are a necessary part of quality health care (Lasiter & Duffy, 2013; Lasiter & McLennon, 2015).
- Nurses have used professional influence to improve the quality of patient care and have provided support for policies that improve health outcomes for populations.
- Nurses bring human and intellectual capital to an institution and use it to advance institutional symbolic and social capital.

The world is ready for nurse professionals who are willing to bypass self-interest and take a strong leadership stance to create a promising future for health care. Nurses are well-positioned to lead the way because they have consistent public support, have in-depth knowledge and know how health care systems work, and possess unspent professional capital. Nurses, however, must be cautious when deciding how to spend professional capital, so that the highly valued relationships that have been developed with patients are veraciously protected.

Sue Lasiter

REFERENCES

American Nurses Association (ANA). (2010a). *Scope and standards of practice.* Silver Spring, MD: Author.

American Nurses Association (ANA). (2010b). *Nursing's social policy statement: The essence of the profession.* Silver Spring, MD: Author.

American Nurses Association (ANA). (2013). *News release: Public ranks nurses as most trusted profession: 11th year in number one slot in gallup poll.* Retrieved May 31,

2013, from http://nursingworld.org/HomepageCategory/NursingInsider/Archive_1/2010-NI/Dec10-NI/Gallup-Poll-Rank-Nurses.html

American Nurses Association (ANA). (2015). *Code for nurses with interpretive statements*. Silver Spring, MD: Author.

Boix, C., & Posner, D. (1998). The origins and political consequences of social capital. *British Journal of Political Science, 28,* 686–693.

Bourdieu, P. (1984). *Distinction: A social critique of the judgement of taste.* Cambridge, MA: Harvard University Press.

Bourdieu, P. (1986). The forms of capital. In J. Richardson (Ed.), *Handbook of theory and research for the sociology of education* (pp. 241–258). New York, NY: Greenwood.

Cashman, S. B., Reidy, P., Cody, K., & Lemay, C. A. (2004). Developing and measuring progress toward collaborative, integrated, interdisciplinary health care teams. *Journal of Interprofessional Care, 18*(2), 183–196.

Casey, K. L. (2008, April). *Defining political capital: A reconsideration of Bourdieu's Interconvertibility Theory.* Paper presented at the Illinois State University Conference for Students of Political Science, Normal, IL.

Clicker, D. S., & Shirey, M. R. (2013). Professional comportment: The missing element in nursing practice. *Nursing Forum, 48*(2), 106–113.

Covell, C. L. (2008). The middle-range theory of nursing intellectual capital. *Journal of Advanced Nursing, 63,* 94–103.

DeFrino, D. T. (2009). A theory of the relational work of nurses. *Research and Theory for Nursing Practice: An International Journal, 23*(4), 294–311.

Drucker, P. F. (1994, November). The age of social transformation. *Atlantic Monthly,* pp. 53–80.

Drucker, P. F. (1999). Knowledge-worker productivity: The biggest challenge. *California Management Review, 41*(2), 79–94.

Duffy, J. (2013). *Quality caring in nursing and health systems: Implications for clinicians, educators, and leaders.* New York, NY: Springer Publishing Company.

Fletcher, S., Berg, A., Simmermann, M., Wuste, K., & Behrens, J. (2007). Nurse–patient interaction and communication: A systematic literature review. *Journal of Public Health, 17*(5), 339–353.

Gallup. (2013). *Honesty/ethics in professions.* Retrieved January 19, 2015, from http://www.gallup.com/poll/1654/honesty-ethicsprofessions.aspx

Herold, D. M., & Fedor, D. B. (2008). The effects of transformational and change leadership on employees' commitment to change: A multilevel study. *Journal of Applied Psychology, 93*(2), 346–357.

Institute for Healthcare Improvement (IHI). (2007). *The Triple Aim: Care, health, and cost.* Retrieved December 27, 2014 from http://www.ihi.org/resources/Pages/Publications/TripleAimCareHealthandCost.aspx

Institute of Medicine (IOM). (2010). *The future of nursing: Leading change, advancing health.* Retrieved from http://www.thefutureofnursing.org/sites/default/files/Future%20of%20Nursing%20Report_0.pdf

Interprofessional Education Collaborative Expert Panel. (2011). *Core competencies for interprofessional collaborative practice: Report of an expert panel.* Washington, DC: Interprofessional Education Collaborative.

Johns Hopkins University School of Nursing and the Berman Institute of Bioethics. (2014). *A blueprint for 21st century nursing ethics: Report of the national nursing summit.* Retrieved November 18, 2014, from http://www.bioethicsinstitute.org/wp-content/uploads/2014/09/Executive_summary.pdf

Kline, T. J., Willness, C., & Ghali, W. A. (2008). Predicting patient complaints in hospital settings. *Quality and Safety in Health Care, 17*(5), 346–350.

Lasiter, S., & Duffy, J. (2013). Older adults' perceptions of feeling safe in urban and rural acute care. *Journal of Nursing Administration, 43*(1), 30–36.

Lasiter, S., & McLennon, S. (2015). Nursing professional capital: A qualitative analysis. *Journal of Nursing Administration, 45*(2), 107–112.

Mazzocco, K., Pettiti, D. B., & Fong, K. T. (2009). Surgical team behaviors and patient outcomes, *American Journal of Surgery, 197*(5), 678–685.

Merton, M. K. (1960). The search for professional status: Sources, costs, and consequences. *American Journal of Nursing, 60*(2), 662–664.

Reeves, S., Zwarenstein, M., Goldman, J., Barr, H., Freeth, D., Hammick, M., & Koppel, I. (2009). Interprofessional education: Effects on professional practice and healthcare outcomes (Review). *Cochrane Database of Systematic Reviews, 2009*(4). doi:10.1002/14651858.CD002213.pub2

Schinkel, W., & Noordegraaf, M. (2011). Professionalism as symbolic capital: Materials for a Bourdieusian theory of professionalism. *Comparative Sociology, 10*(1), 67–96.

Tarlier, D. S. (2004). Beyond caring: The moral and ethical bases of responsive nurse-patient relationship. *Nursing Philosophy, 5*(3), 230–241.

Thistlethwaite, J., & Dallest, K. (2014). Interprofessional teamwork: Still haven't decided what we are educating for? *Medical Education, 48*(6), 556–558.

Wilkinson, T. J., Wade, W. B., & Knock, L. D. (2009). A blueprint to assess professionalism: Results of a systematic review. *Academic Medicine, 84*(5), 551–558.

World Health Organization (WHO). (2010). *Framework for action on interprofessional education and collaborative practice.* Retrieved February 3, 2015 from http://whqlibdoc.who.int/hq/2010/WHO_HRH_HPN_10.3_eng.pdf?ua=1

PART **II**

From Design to Enculturation

Components of Professional Practice Models: Design

Values clarification, theoretical framework, patient care delivery systems, shared leadership, shared governance

By the end of this chapter, readers will be able to:

1. Appreciate the values inherent in professional nursing
2. Choose well-aligned theoretical frameworks that uphold nursing's disciplinary perspective
3. Analyze related elements of patient care delivery systems (PCDSs)
4. Apply principles of shared leadership to the workplace
5. Create a visual representation of a professional practice model (PPM)

NAMING THE VALUES INHERENT IN PROFESSIONAL NURSING

Nursing values connote particular beliefs about professional nursing and establish how one feels about the profession. These work-related values are different from, but related to, those personal values that we use to frame our lives. Work values are a subset of personal values that represent enduring views concerning nursing practice and the profession that shape how nurses conduct themselves, make decisions, and commit to the work.

> In essence, work values are those views of the nursing role that individuals find most important and that serve to motivate and connect nurses to their core principles.

Although nursing values are oftentimes based on individual religious and sociocultural perspectives, as well as on certain life experiences, they are further shaped by education, work experiences, and the context in which one works.

In times of great change or competing priorities (such as integrating a professional practice model [PPM]), or when working with underdeveloped employees, nursing values provide the stability to persevere. In one editorial, the nursing values of human dignity and respect, altruism, social justice, precise care, and appropriate relationships were identified as most typical (Condon & Hegge, 2011). Others have spoken of trust, nearness, sympathy, support, knowledge, and responsibility (Snellman & Gedda, 2012). Still others have identified advocacy, caring, compassion, and excellence as significant nursing values (Watson, 2006). Many of these beliefs are contained in the American Nurses Association (ANA) *Code of Ethics* (2015). Clarity and attention to individual work-related values help raise nurses' awareness, direct their priorities, and enable nurses to make choices. In fact, some have found that when individual work-related values were consistent with role performance, reduced job dissatisfaction, increased motivation, and increased retention followed (Ravari, Bazargan-Hejazi, Ebadi Mirzaei, & Oshvandi, 2013).

> A nursing value system shared among numerous employees links many nurses who work together, impacts system performance, and solidifies nursing's image in an organization.

Shared work-related values facilitate organizational goals by confirming role definitions, establishing appropriate competencies, directing educational activities, enabling teamwork, providing a starting point for change, organizing strategic priorities, and contributing to professional identity. Through shared values, organizations build cultures that contribute to or detract from goals.

> In the context of developing a PPM, clarifying a set of shared values provides the necessary foundation for the PPM's design.

Furthermore, the value set can be used to craft a nursing philosophy that helps explain nursing's shared reflection of its practice, including its contribution to the community served. When aligned with the larger organization's mission, shared professional nursing values position health systems to better actualize the organization's long-term vision.

The process of values clarification involves a brief activity or a set of brief activities that help individuals identify, clarify, and prioritize those beliefs about nursing that are central to them.

> Values-exploration exercises, in which individuals are typically asked to identify and rank order convictions about nursing, provide an opportunity for nurses from distinct areas of a health system to come together and think deeply about nursing, identify its important truths, reflect and consider consequences, and choose those beliefs that fit best with the organization and the community it serves.

Usually, values clarification in nursing requires representatives from multiple areas of a health system to gather in a quiet place for 1 to 2 hours with a facilitator. As an alternative, in a large institution where it is difficult to get many nurses together at one time, scheduling small groups at different times until all have been involved is an option. The key to developing and realizing a common shared vision is to involve as many stakeholders as possible in the process.

The facilitator can be anyone who has some experience with groups and does not necessarily need to be a nurse. Usually, the exercise starts with a question to help identify the main purpose. For example, what do you believe is the ultimate goal of nursing? This question can then be followed by a second one that is more specific such as: How can this goal be achieved? If necessary, other questions can be asked to stimulate more discussion (see Table 4.1).

Table 4.1 Suggested Values-Clarification Questions

- I believe the ultimate purpose of nursing is…
- I believe this purpose can be achieved by…
- I believe patients and families are…
- I believe my role as a nurse is…

Once certain values/beliefs are named, the facilitator can lead a dialogue about them, freely discussing the members' reactions to them, emphasizing that various nurses will react differently.

Second, the facilitator can probe potential organizational consequences of using these values to guide nursing practice by asking questions such as:

- How might these values be viewed by patients, families, other health care workers, or administrators?
- How will other nurses who are not here today view these beliefs about nursing?
- Will other nurses and/or health professionals work with you to uphold these values in practice?
- Can you envision these values in place 50 years from now?

On the other hand, the facilitator can present the group with a prearranged list of nursing values and ask participants to rank order those they feel are most significant. Although efficient, a drawback of this method is the lack of deep reflection on the part of the participant. Using facilitation techniques, such as dialogic conversation, allowing equal voice, paraphrasing and mirroring, drawing people out, deliberate refocusing, and managing group energy ensures a comprehensive and participative process (Kaner, 2014). As specific values are articulated, they are documented and a system of analysis is used to prioritize those with the most significant meaning to the group. For example, the Delphi technique (Dalkey & Helmer, 1963; Dalkey, 1969) can be used to communicate and collate multiple iterative responses and then generate consensus on a final list of nursing values. It is prudent to keep this final list short for ease of comprehension and integration into existing documents. When finalized, the group or groups then disseminate their results to a larger group (sometimes the practice council) for approval and record keeping. See Appendix A for an outline of a values-clarification workshop. The finalized values are then confirmed to others through organization-specific documents such as nursing philosophy statements, commitment declarations, or proclamations of what characterizes nursing in a certain health system. For example, the Advocate Health System in Illinois generated a list of nursing values, labeling them "The Advocate Nurse" to distinguish nursing at this organization. They include:

- Innovation
- Leadership
- Clinical excellence

- Compassion
- Professional growth
- Patient-centered, holistic care

The Advocate Nurse (2014)
Advocate Health System
Chicago, Illinois

ALIGNMENT OF ORGANIZATIONAL MISSION, NURSING VALUES, AND STRATEGIC DIRECTION

Organizational missions vary but they relate to a health system's ultimate purpose (e.g., patient care, research, or education). A mission statement suggests what an organization is, what it does, and, in some cases, where the organization plans to be in the future.

Although work values, in which employees are emotionally invested, illustrate what is important to them, mission statements inform employees of what they should be doing.

For example, a hospital's mission statement might read:

Patients First In Everything We Do. We are sensitive and responsive to the individual needs of our patients and their family members; we are committed to providing quality care to our patients through a highly trained and motivated staff, state-of-the-art equipment, progressive clinical care, and collaborative teamwork; we continuously evaluate and improve our services to meet the needs of our patients and the community we serve; we go the extra mile to serve our customers with kindness, compassion, and respect.

Lowell General Hospital (2015a)
Lowell, Massachusetts

The articulated nursing philosophy (with embedded nursing values), however, states:

At Lowell General Hospital, it is the belief of the professional nursing staff that every individual has the right to be cared for and to receive quality health care. It is the belief of the professional nursing staff that quality nursing practice has its basis in theory validated by evidence-based practice and nursing research. Nursing at Lowell General Hospital is committed to initiate and participate in research in an ongoing effort to define and improve standards of nursing care and to seek new knowledge, innova- tions, and improvements. This dynamic nursing environment en- sures commitment to nursing as a unique profession in making a contribution to the overall health of the patients in our community.

Nursing Philosophy

Lowell General Hospital (2015b)

Lowell, Massachusetts

The values expressed in the nursing philosophy statement suggest patients' rights to quality care, the importance of evidence-based practice (EBP), research and performance improvement, and nursing's contribution to over- all health. And the mission statement clearly outlines the hospital's commit- ment to patients in terms of providing quality and compassionate care.

In a side-by-side comparison of the two statements, consistencies can be identified. In this case, both documents are aligned, allowing for optimal integration of the PPM (see Table 4.2). If, after careful appraisal, however, the mission statement and the articulated nursing values lack congruency, it is important to regroup and consider creating a more consistent set of docu- ments. In most cases, the mission statement cannot be revised and it drives organizational plans, image, and performance.

One approach to resolving inconsistent documents is to take the time to examine the mission statement and selected nursing values together with common everyday nursing tasks. This provides insight into the organiza- tion's workflow that may drive a reiteration of the values. In performing

Table 4.2 Consistency Between Mission Statement and Nursing Values

Mission Statement (Sets Organizational Direction)	Nursing Values (Beliefs)
Patients first; sensitive responsive care	"Patients have a right to be cared for"
Quality care	"Every patient has a right to quality care"
Highly trained staff	"Improve standards of nursing; seek new knowledge, innovation, improvements"
Progressive clinical care	"Commitment to overall health of community"
Continuously evaluate and improve	"Evidence-based practice"
Kindness, compassion, and respect	"Practice based on theory"

this exercise, some health systems find that the complexity of the system may interfere with actualizing the core values. Another alternative is to look for those individuals who best reflect the stated values and then determine whether these employees exhibit behaviors that represent the organization's mission. Any inconsistencies should be addressed. Taking these examples back to the values clarification group and renaming only those core values that are *fundamental* to the organizational mission better positions the health system to realize successful PPM integration.

Aligning the organizational mission and core nursing values must occur at a variety of levels across a health system, requiring strong leadership and ongoing monitoring. Understanding and recognizing this important relationship, taking a "big picture" view with the ability to appreciate many different perspectives, being able to identify common themes, make decisions despite political agendas, and consider implications of actions are valuable leadership qualities.

> Proper alignment of the organizational mission and nursing values informs the choice of theoretical foundation, which is the way nursing work will be framed.

CHOOSING A THEORETICAL FRAMEWORK

A theoretical foundation strengthens nursing practice by providing parameters for that practice, a common disciplinary language, a basis for research, guidance for specific interventions, and the foundation for advancement systems (Smith & Parker, 2015). Choosing or developing a framework that is consistent with stated nursing values is crucial. Furthermore, the framework makes explicit what is implied by the values statement and unifies nursing practice across a health system.

> Choosing a theoretical framework is best accomplished by a group of practicing clinicians (typically members of a practice council) for whom the ultimate framework will demand action.

Grounded by the organizational mission statement and nursing values, a review of several existing theories, including the authors' assumptions, major concepts, and relationships, should proceed with special attention to the population served. Acquiring and reading the authors' primary works and using an acceptable evaluation system (e.g., criteria for evaluation of theory; Fawcett, 2005; Chinn & Kramer, 2011) to evaluate the theories is a good process for choosing one that best represents a good fit with the organization's mission, nursing values, and the particular theory (Table 4.3).

> When evaluating a theory for PPM inclusion, it is especially important to analyze whether the concepts are understandable, whether the theory is practical for the context, and whether it is significant for the population being served. Additionally, it is helpful to consider whether the theory has been used in research, whether there are operational definitions for its concepts, and whether it has been adopted by other health systems.

Although many organizations choose to adopt an existing nursing theory, several organizations have developed their own foundational principles to guide nursing practice. For example, Banner Health System developed a conceptual framework starting with broad guiding principles and assumptions and continuing with contributions to patients, the profession, and society (Mensik, Martin, Scott, & Horton, 2011).

Whether choosing an existing model or developing one's own, the selection should be precise, with multiple views from across the organization considered. Edmundson (2012) details the process used at one pediatric hospital using a representative selection team, in-depth readings, multiple meetings, and communications with other health systems.

> The final result of selecting and acknowledging a theoretical foundation for nursing that is consistent with the organizational mission and contemporary nursing values positions a health system to consider how nursing work will be arranged to deliver care that embodies that foundation, that is, its patient care delivery system (PCDS).

Table 4.3 Considerations for Choosing a Nursing Theoretical Framework

- Consistency with organizational nursing values
- Consideration of population served
- Clear, understandable concepts
- Ease of translation to practice
- Measurable tools available
- Evidence (research) of its benefits
- Successful use by other health systems

THE PATIENT CARE DELIVERY SYSTEM

The term *patient care delivery system*, refers to how care is organized and coordinated in health systems. More specific, it describes the approach to care delivery, the skill sets required, authority and accountability for decision making and resultant patient outcomes, how multiple health care workers communicate and coordinate care, environmental artifacts and equipment that support the process, and what resources are required. Traditionally, PCDSs referred to the acute care environment and were associated with nursing and ancillary staff (e.g., team nursing, functional nursing, total patient care, primary nursing). Later, although still referring to nursing in the acute care environment, systems, such as the partnership model, sometimes referred to as coprimary nursing, were designed to make more efficient use of the RN (Marquis & Huston, 2000).

In the partnership model the RN is partnered with a licensed practical nurse (LPN) or an unlicensed assistive personnel (UAP), and the pair work together consistently to care for an assigned group of patients. Another system, modular nursing, calls for a smaller group of staff providing care for a smaller group of patients. The goal of this model was to increase the involvement of the RN in planning and coordinating care and maximize communication among team members (Anderson & Hughes, 1993).

Case management is another care delivery system; in the case management system an RN coordinates the patient's care throughout the course of an illness. Case management is generally used for chronically ill, seriously ill or injured, and long-term, high-cost cases. In this system of care, because of the chronic, long-term nature of the patient population, the role of the RN is much broader than a specific unit and today this model is used by both health systems and most major health insurance companies. Health systems use case management to augment unit-based systems and insurance companies use it to manage the use (and ultimately costs) of health care services for their clients.

The ANA defines *nursing case management* as

a dynamic and systematic collaborative approach to providing and coordinating health care services to a defined population. It is a participative process to identify and facilitate options and services for meeting individuals' health needs, while decreasing fragmentation and duplication of care and enhancing quality, cost-effective clinical outcomes. The framework for nursing care management includes five components: assessment, planning, implementation, evaluation, and interaction.

(Llewellyn & Leonard, 2009, p. 12)

Although case management is known as a form of patient care delivery for one site, in today's remodeled health system, the term *patient care delivery system* has taken on a broader meaning, one that crosses health care settings, such as acute hospital care, to include larger integrated arrangements that extend into the community, align multiple health care providers, and are coordinated through health information systems. For example, the patient-centered medical home includes patient-centered, team-based care that is coordinated across traditional health care system boundaries, with enhanced access using alternative methods of communication (e.g., remote monitoring, electronic reminders, and networked electronic health records), and a systems-based approach to quality and safety (Scholle, Torda, Peikes, Han, & Genevro, 2010).

Whereas the care team traditionally included RNs, LPNs, and nursing assistants (NAs), current care teams include all relevant health care providers, including the family, whose collective efforts result in optimal care. Of course, health systems also design their own PCDSs. For example, at MD Anderson Cancer Center in Houston, Texas, a primary team approach was designed that incorporates a microsystem of nurses and other health team members who cooperatively and consistently provide care to a small group of patients. To facilitate the primary team, a master's-prepared nurse supports continuity and coordination among the members, builds relationships, uses outcomes data to expedite practice changes, and coaches and develops primary team members (Duffy, 2013). Although each of these approaches offers benefits and challenges, both the traditional and newer approaches to patient care delivery lack good evidence of their value (e.g., clinical, experiential, and cost outcomes). It is imperative that PCDSs be evaluated to determine their ultimate value.

> Designing a PCDS takes into consideration the population served; a set of guiding principles; and the roles, responsibilities, and relationships of care providers involved, including their authority for decision making, the infrastructure, and the environment. Its ultimate goal is to foster high-value health care for patients and families, but also to define the authority, accountability, and autonomy for clinical decision making and outcomes.

As such, a better grasp of the tasks and roles of providers, as well as patient outcomes, results. Designing the PCDS is best accomplished through a group process approach with all levels of professional nursing involved. In other words, over a series of meetings, a facilitator works with a group of staff nurses, nurse leaders, nurse educators, and others to develop the blueprint for how nursing care (as defined by the mission/values and theoretical framework) will be delivered. Whether adopting an existing PCDS or designing one specific to an institution, a well-defined series of activities enables appropriate alignment with the values and beliefs that formed the foundation of the PPM (see Table 4.4).

First, a thorough understanding of the population served is essential. Understanding patients' and families' needs and preferences is a hallmark of patient-centered care (Institute of Medicine [IOM] Committee on Quality of Health Care in America, 2001) and is an overriding theme in today's health system.

Obtaining feedback from patients on those symptoms that truly limit their lives (versus those health providers concentrate on), exploring the meaning of their illnesses, identifying their health goals, understanding their unique perspectives about health and health care (e.g., how do they want to participate and make decisions?), and, in general, grasping what matters to them facilitates patient centeredness.

Being aware of these perspectives enables analysis of the facility and the staff who best can provide these services, assurance that the overall experience of care is optimal, enables safety, and sets up the conditions for transparent communication between patients and health care providers. In this way, a true emphasis on patients as partners versus patients as passive recipients is upheld. As the population becomes better known, designers can then respond to their needs and preferences by reviewing the mission/values and nursing theoretical framework, already defined, to develop a set of guiding principles that will drive the type of nursing care that will be delivered.

Table 4.4 Activities Used to Design a Patient Care Delivery System

- Assemble appropriate group of diverse stakeholders; assign facilitator
- Reflect on population served and their unique needs
- Develop a list of guiding principles
- Define employee roles, work responsibilities, and relationships among care providers (revise job descriptions, assign authority for decision making and documentation as needed)
- Consider infrastructure (resources, assignment patterns, skill mix, supplies and equipment, communication systems)
- Describe environmental features supporting nursing practice
- Include special theoretically based factors (e.g., nursing interventions, interprofessional collaboration, professional development)

Guiding principles are more explicit than values or beliefs and are meant to guide nursing *actions* in the context of a specific health system and a specific patient population. In essence, they set the norms or rules that represent what actions are desired and affirm the professional code of conduct. Guiding principles are intended to proactively direct the professional practice of nursing (set the standard for everyday nursing practice in a health system) and to inform nursing stakeholders (patients, families, other health professionals) about the principles they can expect will be upheld. Guiding principles generally cover all departments of nursing in a health system, with any exceptions documented and rationales provided. Guiding principles can oftentimes overlap; thus, professional nurses must use their judgment and expert knowledge of patients and families to determine the appropriate response in a given situation. If a course of action is unclear, soliciting the advice of fellow nursing professionals or leadership about how to resolve the problem before deciding how to proceed is warranted. Finally, guiding principles are part of an evolving process of self-examination by professional nurses. They should be revisited and examined for possible review and revision on a regular basis—at least every 3 years. An example of guiding principles, drawn from a hospital in the suburban Washington, DC, area follows (Duffy, 2009; Duffy, Baldwin, & Mastorovich, 2007):

- The patient/family is the authority for care received, not the clinician or the institution
- Patients and families are entitled to caring relationships
- Patients see a limited number of faces while hospitalized
- Nurses are knowledge workers who are continuously learning; accessing knowledge is a required nursing behavior
- The patient–nurse relationship informs practice
- The core of nursing work is caring
- Time spent interacting with patients and families is expected, valued, and rewarded
- Collaborative relationships with the health care team are not optional; they are mandatory
- Responsibility for caring–healing–protective environments rests on all of us

Next, using the mission/values and theoretical framework, supported by professional standards, nurse practice acts, and guiding principles, clearly defining the role of the professional nurse in light of expressed patient needs is paramount. Examining the professional nurse job description and adjusting the associated behaviors to more clearly represent the chosen nursing values and theoretical framework prevents role ambiguity and provides the basis for UAP performance summaries. Such clarity lays the groundwork for performance and ensures that the workforce understands its scope of practice, including accountability for clinical decisions and patient outcomes. This activity leads to the specification of clinical work processes (e.g., physical assessment, evaluation of learning needs and patient education, establishing therapeutic relationships, hygiene practices, developing and revising the plan of care, collaboration with physicians and other care providers), detailing who does what, how and when the work is conducted, and documentation practices (e.g., clinical workflow).

> Clinical workflow encompasses all those actions and interactions clinicians utilize to meet the needs of patients and families and is best performed when the responsibilities of employees are transparently documented.

Next, carefully describe the infrastructure required to support the work, such as the resources required (e.g., numbers of employees, skill mix, assignment plans, supplies and equipment), communication patterns (e.g., information systems used, shift report and handoffs procedures), and leadership. Based on patient and family care needs and consistent with the description of professional nursing, the PCDS design team can then plan for required personnel and materials needed. At this point, it is essential to consider how professional nursing has been defined by the chosen theoretical framework, so that appropriate numbers and types of personnel can be assigned. Additionally, as evidence clearly points to the relationship between appropriate nurse staffing and safe patient outcomes (Aiken Clarke, Sloane, Sochalski, & Silber, 2002; Estabrooks, Midodzi, Cummings, Ricker, & Giovannetti, 2005; McHugh, Berez, & Small, 2013; Needleman, Buerhaus, Mattke, Stewart, & Zelevinsky, 2002; Rafferty et al., 2007; Tourangeau, Cranley, & Jeffs, 2006; Tourangeau et al., 2007), those designing PCDSs must use these important findings to ensure patient safety as well as to consider individual employee workload. Optimal nurse staffing plans recognize unique departmental factors, specific times of day that are especially demanding (such as during patient admissions and discharges), and include consideration of patient age, psychosociocultural characteristics, acuity, use of UAP, specialized equipment or protocols, and the skills, education, and training of employees

(Serratt, Myer, & Chapman, 2014). Working through such factors eventually helps achieve consensus regarding who and how decisions for patient assignments are to be made.

In addition to the numbers and types of employees required, how assignments are made to ensure consistency and coordination of services is crucial. Finally, using the PPM definition of professional nursing, how supplies and equipment are made available, kept in working order, and arranged to meet the needs of patients and families should be specified.

Communication patterns that describe how employees give and receive information to ensure safe coordination of services is also part of the PCDS. These patterns include face-to-face, electronic, written, telephonic, and all other means used to enable accurate and timely information flow. Responsibility and accountability for specific communication practices (such as shift reports, staff meetings) should be documented, thorough, and clear.

The next step in defining the PCDS includes specific environmental features that support the work, such as safety equipment, bulletin boards, waiting rooms, images, lighting, noise, smells, general cleanliness and aesthetics, air flow, educational materials, respect for patient confidentiality and privacy, policies and procedures, human resources policies, and departmental climate. Although not directly tied to patient care, these components of the care delivery system influence how well and efficiently the work of nursing is accomplished. Thus, the design team should consider their influence as the PCDS is being created.

Finally, because some theoretical notions of nursing are more focused than others, many designers have included particular nursing interventions in the PCDS that represent the nursing theoretical stance adopted. For example, one aspect of Watson's caring theory (Watson, 2012) specifies "transpersonal caring moments" during which persons relate in meaningful, authentic, and intentional ways. To facilitate this form of nursing practice, some organizations have embedded forced intentional interactions into the daily workflow of professional nurses. Other aspects of current professional practice have also been included in modern PCDSs. For example, how care providers receive ongoing professional development, participate in collaborative practice, or enact departmental-level leadership is frequently part of the PCDS.

Using a clearly delineated approach that remains consistent to the underlying nursing values and theoretical framework ensures a well-aligned PCDS. The final PCDS should clarify and facilitate daily clinical workflow and inform the practice of other health personnel who support nursing.

GOVERNANCE AND SHARED LEADERSHIP

Governance in an organization refers to the mechanisms that organizations deploy to influence members' behaviors such that organizational outcomes are met in a socially acceptable manner (Filatotchev & Makajima, 2014). In essence, governance is about the structure and relationships that allocate power in an organization. Governance implies decision making, authority, stewardship, and control processes that determine organizational direction and eventual achievement of goals. Because employees at all levels within organizations are individuals with unique values, preferences, knowledge, and interests, effective governance typically includes rules, checks, and balances intended to limit or prevent the tension between individual self-interests and broader organizational goals. In health care, good governance is central to high performance.

The World Health Organization views governance in health care delivery as a function of standards, information, incentives, and accountability (Lewis & Petterson, 2009). Standards, when transparent, inform performance such that acceptable behaviors and levels of achievement can be established. Incentives are motivating factors that encourage and reward behaviors, whereas accurate and timely information flow provides clarity and feedback. Finally, and probably most important, governance ensures accountability such that individuals at all levels of an organization are held responsible for processes and outcomes and appropriate sanctions are imposed when necessary.

To fulfill these functions, governance structures routinely monitor resources (budget, payroll irregularities, purchasing practices), providers (credentials, absenteeism, performance, engagement), system performance (length of stay, occupancy rates, adverse outcomes), and perceptions (satisfaction, experience). Past systems of governance relied on a centralized, hierarchical leadership approach, whereas more modern systems use a distributed, relational method that emphasizes teamwork, collegiality, collaboration, and partnering among leadership, employees, and stakeholders, also known as shared leadership.

Shared leadership, practiced for centuries in some governments, churches, and academic organizations (Sally, 2002), emphasizes "dynamic and influential processes among individuals in groups for which the objective is to lead one another to the achievement of group or organizational goals or both. This influence process often involves peer, or lateral, influence and at other times involves upward or downward hierarchical influence" (Pearce & Conger, 2003, p. 1), signifying the ongoing evolution of this process. This definition differs from traditional, tiered, position-based leadership and is more consistent with complexity theory and relational leadership principles. As Goldsmith (2010) contends, shared leadership maximizes talent such that employees are empowered by the opportunity to guide the direction of their own practice (area of expertise). This form of leadership emphasizes leaders as facilitators or coaches versus the sources of authority, encouraging reciprocal relationships in which team members share purposes, offer social support, and lend voice to decisions (Carson, Tesluk, & Marrone, 2007). Prerequisites to shared leadership include those indicated in Table 4.5.

Although scientific data on the benefits of shared leadership are scant, anecdotal evidence of better decision making and increased creativity and team effectiveness has been documented (Avolio, Walumbwa, & Weber, 2009).

> Whereas shared leadership is a characteristic that enables members to engage in certain behaviors that complement each other, increasing the probability of team progress toward desired goals, shared governance refers to the actual system for decision making that empowers employees to oversee their practice.

This has been an important empowering tool for professional nurses since the late 1980s and is included in the American Nurses Credentialing Center (ANCC; 2013) Magnet® criteria as structural empowerment.

Descriptions of shared governance have changed over the years from an accountability-based system for professional staff (O'Grady, 1987), to dynamic, participatory, decision-making systems that regulate professional nurses' practice (Lovan, Shaffer, & Murray, 2004), to evolutionary processes that advance over time (Meyers & Costanzo, 2015). Shared governance assumes autonomy and accountability for professional practice, and allows for nursing empowerment and collaboration in decisions that affect individual patient care, the more general practice environment, and group

Table 4.5 Shared Leadership Role Responsibilities

- Commitment of senior leadership
- Upfront investment of time (to educate members and plan actions)
- Fundamental management practices in place (supervision, communication mechanisms, and decision-making rules)
- Engagement and accountability

Adapted from Allison, Misra, and Perry (2014).

governance (Burnhope & Edmonstone, 2003). Shared governance also implies working with other disciplines for the good of the patient and continuously improving nursing practice.

Because nurses are the largest group of employees in a health system, they share a large proportion of the budget and, at the same time, are essential to the quality (value) of the services a health system delivers. In this era of health care transformation, it is essential to earn and maintain the trust of the workforce, promote a culture of trust and accountability, and advance cohesive goals. Thus, shared governance as one component of the overall PPM must be a robust system of decision making, monitoring, and employing safeguards that ensure the health of the community served. According to O'Grady (2001), shared governance systems are founded on four principles: partnership, equity, accountability, and ownership.

Partnership includes honoring the links that providers have with patients and families, communities, suppliers, leadership, and regulators. Equity ensures diversity of services and employees to ensure maximum participation and decision making, whereas accountability ensures responsibilities are appropriately carried out. Finally, ownership implies that everyone is essential to the business.

Using the mission/values, nursing theoretical framework, and PCDS, designing the system for shared governance includes:

- Deciding on the right numbers and levels of participants and committee structure
- Ensuring diversity of employees involved (service area, gender, work experience, etc.)
- Appointment of members (including terms of appointment)
- A detailed and explicit process (or a set of rules, bylaws, charter) for maximizing meetings and team processes
- Ensuring engagement through advance preparation (e.g., focused meeting agendas, expected preparation for meetings), attendance alternatives
- Facilitative leadership
- Effective communication, including electronic means
- Resource support (a budget)
- A system for evaluation (mini evaluations of meetings, attendance and record keeping, annual reports, evaluation of members, overall evaluation)

There are multiple examples in the literature of shared governance systems that include committees or councils representing important aspects of the nursing profession, such as practice or performance improvement councils, with associated bylaws detailing communication and control mechanisms. Some large health organizations actually have a nursing congress with elected representatives, whereas in academia a faculty senate model is often used. Of importance is the appropriate size of the shared governance system for the organization (i.e., number of councils or committees and appropriate representation); their relationships to those on the front lines, other health professionals, and patients/families; *and* the processes for decision making so that practice expertise is preserved.

Some specific examples of activities that professional nurses engage in with established shared governance systems include:

- Create, define, approve, and evaluate nursing practice standards, policies, and procedures
- Participate in continuous improvement, peer review, and professional development
- Collaborate with community representatives and key stakeholders to improve the image of nursing
- Collaborate with others in the organization to maximize the practice environment for excellent care delivery

As the workforce emerges, members of shared governance committees assume increasing responsibility for their practice, shifting the power base to those clinicians who are actually providing care. Literature has shown that shared governance structures improve nurses' attitudes toward the work environment, improve the climate for innovation and change, enhance nursing work satisfaction and productivity, increase awareness among physicians and other health professionals of nursing's decision-making skills, and provide recognition for nursing's contribution to patient outcomes (Barden, Quinn, Donahue, & Fitzpatrick, 2011).

RECOGNITION AND REWARDS

Recognizing and rewarding professional nurses is difficult. On the one hand, professional nurses commit to quality patient care upon graduation (usually by reciting an oath); but on the other hand, as humans, recognition meets the fundamental human need for belonging and esteem (Maslow, 1943, 1954). Furthermore, *meaningful* recognition of one's work contributions is tied to personal and professional development (AACN, 2005). For example, *meaningful* recognition has been positively correlated with psychological capital (hope, optimism, self-efficacy, and resilience; Avolio & Luthans, 2006;

Froman, 2010; Luthans, Avey, Avolio, & Peterson, 2010; Luthans & Youssef, 2004), an important workplace characteristic (Laschinger & Fida, 2014). It has also been associated with nurse retention and engagement (Carter & Tourangeau, 2012; Chan & Morrison, 2000), job embeddedness (Bargagliotti, 2012), and workgroup cohesion (Cowden & Cummings, 2012). Furthermore, meaningful recognition provides a vehicle for naming the tangibles associated with patient care (Lefton, 2012) and shaping a culture of appreciation in which conversations about personal issues are allowed, employee opinions are sought, and career objectives can mature (Riordan, 2013).

Recognizing exceptional behavior reinforces and rewards those important professional nursing behaviors envisioned by the PPM, giving life and connection to the underlying nursing values.

Of note is the word *meaningful*. In reference to work recognition, *meaningful* connotes acknowledging behaviors and their impact on others, ensuring the feedback is relevant to the recognized situation and is equal to the person's contribution (AACN, 2005). Moreover, providing meaningful recognition sends the message to employees that they matter in a system that seems ostensibly large and confusing. Such feedback is best provided by considering first who the employee would most want to convey the feedback, what the employee truly values, the time and place to express the recognition (e.g., some individuals enjoy public displays whereas others are more private), and finally, how the feedback links to organizational purpose (in this case to the PPM; Nelson & Spitzer, 2003).

Used effectively, recognition and reinforcement (rewards), help strengthen the evolving PPM by first noticing and then acknowledging important nursing actions, ultimately influencing organizational purpose.

Of course, properly aligning nursing actions to be recognized and rewarded with the articulated nursing values and theoretical framework specified in the PPM is paramount. Of importance is noticing the valuable work immediately, specificity of the recognized behavior, equity across the organization, and the consistency with which the recognition is applied across a health system.

Many health systems have both formal recognition programs (hospital-wide events) that are structured, budgeted for, and align well with the organization's goals and values—for example, annual employee appreciation awards for years of service—as well as informal recognition programs. Informal, more local recognition, tends to consist of spontaneous, leader-defined events that are not usually measured or tracked. This informal day-to-day recognition seems to be the most powerful, particularly when the person is noticed by name and the leader expresses how the associated action made him or her feel in light of the value it added to the organization. Some view this combination approach of both formal and informal recognition as most beneficial because it provides whole-system and departmental ownership.

Formal recognition programs are usually budgeted and managed centrally and are associated with specific goals. For example, in an organization that values loyalty, recognizing years of service would be important, whereas those who want to motivate performance may recognize certain employee actions.

> In this instance, when a PPM is evolving and plans for integration are in process, it would be important to recognize behaviors that reveal acquisition of new knowledge, increased professionalism, optimism for the future, inspiration, and teamwork, as well as behaviors that reflect specific components of the model.

The types of awards will vary by institution but typically, gift certificates, cash, continuing-education conferences, food, paid time off, and institution-specific artifacts are used. Most important is the genuineness and personalized perspective of the process. Other mechanisms for incentivizing behavior include progression or development programs.

Clinical advancement programs (or clinical ladders), used for over 30 years to reward excellence in clinical practice, have shown limited results (Winslow et al., 2011). In fact, despite their goal to improve clinical nurses' job satisfaction and turnover, participation rates in these programs have varied (Riley, Rolband, James, & Norton, 2009; Winslow et al., 2011). Ensuring that clinical advancement programs are relevant and tied to the PPM is paramount. For example, Owens and Cleaves (2012) describe the update of a clinical advancement program that includes four levels of practice framed by the organization's nursing philosophy and includes clinical nurses' key responsibilities as well as a salaried payment scheme.

Organization-sponsored networking events and participation/election to national nursing organization committees, mentoring programs, opportunities to participate on education or research teams, supporting clinical

nurses for national awards, and financial support for formal education programs all offer clinical nurses occasions for celebration. Praising professional
achievements outside the organization that advance the profession adds
meaning to the workplace that is invaluable.

TYING IT ALL TOGETHER

The PPM is a culmination of blending all identified components (mission/
values, theoretical framework, PCDS, shared governance, recognition/
rewards) into one prototype that conceptualizes how the model will function
in a given health system. Such an illustration clarifies important model concepts and describes what professional nurses will do with the model. Many
organizations design a diagram to depict the model concepts and the relationships among them. Envisioning it as a whole enables *use* of the model by
expressing what concepts employees must focus on and how these relate to
organizational goals. As a result, the model should be easier to understand
in the context of a unique health system and showcase what is most relevant to professional nursing work. Commonalities of nursing work across a
health system that confirm consistencies of practice can be readily visualized
in such a diagram. The representation also creates a starting point for PPM
language and can be applied in training and orientation sessions, marketing
materials, and continuing-education programs.

PPM diagrams often instill pride and motivation in some employees by visually
expressing the product of their thoughtful work; occasionally, this conveys
a message of a unifying brand signaling an identity in professional nursing
practice that better positions nursing within a specific health system.

Finally, the choice of PPM diagram type (e.g., two- or three-dimensional,
colors, etc.) is a function of users' preferences and funding, but should be
simple and translatable to the bedside.

SUMMARY

In this chapter, work-related values and their ties to organizational goals
were described. The process of values clarification was offered as a means to
prioritize those important beliefs. Consistency between nursing values and
a health system's mission was examined in light of PPM design. Choosing

a theoretical framework to guide nursing practice is best accomplished by a diverse group of nurses (many of whom are clinical nurses) who examine the literature and other organizations and make careful decisions that are consistent with organizational and nursing values. This process facilitates the proper identification and application of a PCDS that fits with the idealized nursing values and exists with a certain context. Considering the population served, using a set of guiding principles, including the infrastructure and environment, a PCDS can be designed that appropriately operationalizes daily workflow. Seeking to monitor and improve professional practice, using shared leadership and governance system for decision making was explained. Finally, a system of meaningful recognition and rewards was introduced to further advance professional practice. Unifying the component parts and formalizing the PPM through a visual representation enhances how the model will be used in a specific health system.

REFLECTIVE APPLICATIONS

For Students

1. What values frame your notion of professional nursing? What about your peers?
2. Find the mission statement of your school. What does it suggest about your program?
3. What artifacts from the environment of the school support the mission statement? Provide examples.
4. Examine the nursing theory page at the Hahn School of Nursing and Health Science or at Clayton State University. What nursing theory best articulates your nursing values? Why? What are its major concepts? How do you think it can best be applied in the clinical setting?
5. Explain care management.
6. Is there a student government system for decision making at your school? Are you an active member? Why or why not?
7. What meaningful awards are offered to students in your school? How do they advance academic behavior?

For Clinical Nurses

1. What values/beliefs best describe your notions of nursing? Why?
2. What is the mission statement of your organization? Where did you find it? What does it suggest about your work? How does it articulate with nursing practice?

3. What theoretical framework guides practice at your organization? How was it chosen? Were you involved? How long has it been in place? Is it still relevant? What are its major concepts?

4. What type of PCDS is used at your organization? How do you know? How does it support/not support the chosen theoretical framework? What is the role of the RN in this system? What is the role of UAP? Are these roles carried out as identified? Why or why not?

5. How does the PCDS drive staffing schedules and assignments?

6. How does the PCDS describe communication and the work environment?

7. Is there a shared governance structure for decision making at your organization? How does it work? Are you involved? Why or why not? What can be done to improve participation in shared governance?

8. What meaningful awards are offered to clinical nurses at your organization? How do they advance professional behavior?

9. Does your organization have a nursing philosophy and a PPM diagram? Where are they kept? Can you describe the PPM diagram to a family member such that he or she understands what nursing does in your organization?

For Nurse Leaders

1. What values/beliefs best describe your notions of nursing? Why?

2. How have shared nursing values been identified and prioritized at your organization? What is your role in this?

3. How does the organizational mission statement "fit" with your nursing values? Or does it? What about shared nursing values? What does the mission statement suggest about the nature of nursing work? How does it align with current nursing practice?

4. What theoretical framework drives nursing practice at your organization? How was it chosen? Is it relevant? How do *you* model the framework?

5. What type of PCDS is used at your organization? How was it developed? How does it support/not support the chosen theoretical framework? Are the roles of employees clear in this system? Are these roles carried out as identified? Why or why not?

6. How does the PCDS drive staffing schedules and assignments?

7. How does the PCDS describe communication and the work environment?

8. How do you ensure that the PCDS allows for collaborative interprofessional practice? How is the PCDS evaluated and improved?

9. Is the shared governance structure for decision making at your organization working? How do you know? Are you involved? Why or why not? What can be done to improve shared governance?

10. What meaningful awards are offered to clinical nurses and nurse managers at your organization? How do they reflect the idealized PPM? Should they be changed?

11. How long ago did your organization develop a nursing philosophy? How about a PPM diagram? Where are they kept? Are they relevant? Do clinical nurses use the PPM diagram to describe professional practice?

For Nurse Educators

1. What values/beliefs best describe your notions of nursing? Why?

2. How have shared nursing values been identified and prioritized at your organization? What is your role in this?

3. How does the organizational mission statement "fit" with your nursing values? Or does it? What about shared nursing values? What does the mission statement suggest about the nature of academic work? How does it align with current academic practice?

4. Is nursing theory considered an important course at the undergraduate level? How do undergraduate students learn about nursing theories as a guide to practice? What could you do to advance this?

5. What teaching strategies can be used to help undergraduate/graduate students learn about PCDSs? What about relevant assignments for clarifying and understanding this important work-related concept?

6. Is the shared governance structure for decision making at your organization working? How do you know? Are you involved? Why or why not? What can be done to improve shared governance?

7. What meaningful awards are offered to students and faculty at your organization? How do they reflect the mission/vision? Should they be changed?

8. Do you have a written nursing philosophy? How long ago was it developed? Where is it kept? Is it relevant? Do students refer to the nursing philosophy in their coursework?

9. How do *you* facilitate student identification of nursing values? Does it work? Is it done more than once in the program?

10. What aspects of this chapter have the most implications for education?

11. Are PCDSs and shared governance "taught" in your curriculum? Why or why not?

Development of a nursing professional practice model (PPM) is a complex process that is multilayered, iterative in nature, and the result of synergies that exist between the PPM and each of its components. As a result, the PPM is far more than the sum of its parts. The evolution of our organization's PPM illustrates this complexity. The interplay between developing the PCDS as a critical component of the PPM and simultaneously revising the PPM is described.

The PPM reflects the full range of our nursing vision and values, our institutional mission and vision, and the foundational theoretical framework that supports these values (see Figure 4.1).

The MD Anderson Nursing PPM is based on the Quality-Caring Model© (QCM; Duffy, 2013). At the core of the model, relationship-centered caring is presented as the desired outcome of interactions that occur between the professional nurse caregiver and:

- The interprofessional team
- The community
- The patient and family
- The "self"

The core is surrounded by five hands representing the key components of the PPM: professional values, professional recognition, professional partnerships, shared governance, and patient care delivery. The five components are enclosed within the ring of the QCM's eight caring factors. The outer ring represents the institutional core values.

As a team from our Nursing Practice Congress was designing the revised PPM, another team was designing our PCDS: Primary Team Nursing (PTN). A guiding principle used in the design of PTN included the primacy of relationship-centered caring among members of the nursing team and also between the nursing team and patients/families, the community, and colleagues. The formation of microsystem teams promulgates relationship-centered caring as small numbers of team members consistently partner in the care given to a specific group of patients.

The professional values of the PPM include autonomy, accountability, and excellence in practice. These values were also central in defining the roles of nursing team members in PTN. One of the aims of PTN was to

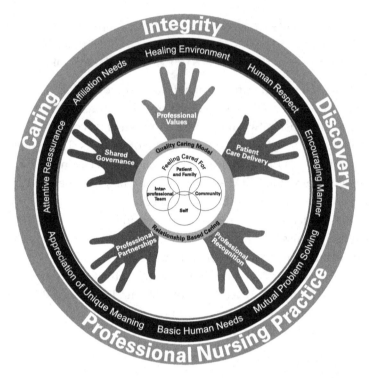

Figure 4.1 MD Anderson Nursing Professional Practice Model. Used with permission.

promote a professional practice group with collective accountability for outcomes of care they delivered.

The eight caring factors of the QCM provided the PTN delivery system with a framework for interaction and building caring relationships. These caring factors are applicable in interactions not only with patients and family members, but also with fellow nursing team members, interprofessional colleagues, and between nursing leaders and their staff members.

Using these tools, we were able to achieve synergy between the PPM and the design of the PCDS, Primary Team Nursing. The outcome—mutually aligned components of the PPM—enhanced successful implementation.

Barbara Summers

REFERENCES

Advocate Health System. (2014). *The advocate nurse*. Minutes of the 2014 Annual Nursing Research Conference. Chicago, IL.

Aiken, L., Clarke, S., Sloane, D., Sochalski, J., & Silber, J. (2002). Hospital nurse staffing and patient mortality, nurse burnout, and job dissatisfaction. *Journal of the American Medical Association, 288*(22), 2948–2954.

American Association of Critical-Care Nurses. (2005). *AACN standards for establishing and sustaining healthy work environments: A journey to excellence.* Retrieved from http://ajcc.aacnjournals.org/content/14/3/187.full.pdfMeaningful recognition

American Nurses Association. (2015). *Code of ethics for nurses with interpretative statements.* Silver Spring, MD: Author.

American Nurses Credentialing Center. (2013). *2014 Magnet® application manual.* Silver Spring, MD: Author.

Anderson, C. L., & Hughes, E. (1993). Implementing modular nursing in a long-term care facility. *Journal of Nursing Administration, 23*(6), 29–35.

Avolio, B. J., Walumbwa, F. O., & Weber, T. J. (2009). Leadership: Current theories, research, and future directions. *Annual Review of Psychology, 60,* 421–449.

Barden, A. M., Quinn, M. T., Donahue, M., & Fitzpatrick, J. J. (2011). Shared governance and empowerment in registered nurse work in a hospital setting. *Nursing Administration Quarterly, 35*(3), 212–218.

Bargagliotti, L. A. (2012). Work engagement in nursing: A concept analysis. *Journal of Advanced Nursing, 68*(6), 1414–1428.

Burnhope, C., & Edmonstone, J. (2003). "Feel the fear and do it anyway": The hard business of developing shared governance. *Journal of Nursing Management, 11,* 147–157.

Carson, J. B., Tesluk, P. E., & Marrone, J. A. (2007). Shared leadership in teams: An investigation of antecedent conditions and performance. *Academy of Management, 50,* 1217–1234.

Carter, M. R., & Tourangeau, A. E. (2012). Staying in nursing: What factors determine whether nurses intend to remain employed? *Journal of Advanced Nursing, 68*(7), 1589–1600.

Chan, E., & Morrison, P. (2000). Factors influencing the retention and turnover intentions of registered nurses in a Singapore hospital. *Nursing and Health Sciences, 2*(2), 113–121.

Chinn, P., & Kramer, M. (2011). *Integrated theory and knowledge development in nursing* (8th ed.). St. Louis, MO: Mosby.

Condon, B. B., & Hegge, M. (2011). Human dignity: A cornerstone of doctoral education in nursing. *Nursing Science Quarterly, 24*(3), 209–214.

Cowden, T. L., & Cummings, G. C. (2012). Nursing theory and concept development: A theoretical model of clinical nurses' intentions to stay in their current positions. *Journal of Advanced Nursing, 68*(7), 1646–1657.

Dalkey, N. C. (1969). An experimental study of group opinion. *Futures, 1*(5), 408–426.

Dalkey, N. C., & Helmer, O. (1963). An experimental application of the Delphi method to the use of experts. *Management Science, 9*(3), 458–467.

Duffy, J. R. (2009). *Quality caring in nursing: Applying theory to clinical practice, education, and leadership.* New York, NY: Springer Publishing Company.

Duffy, J. R. (2013). *Quality caring in nursing and health systems*. New York, NY: Springer Publishing Company.

Duffy, J. R., Baldwin, J., & Mastorovich, M. J. (2007). Using the quality-caring model to organize patient care. *Journal of Nursing Administration, 37*(12), 546–551.

Edmundson, E. (2012). The quality caring nursing model: A journey to selection and implementation. *Journal of Pediatric Nursing: Nursing Care of Children and Families, 27*(4), 411–415.

Estabrooks, C., Midodzi, W., Cummings, G., Ricker, K., & Giovannetti, P. (2005). Impact of hospital characteristics on 30-day mortality. *Nursing Research, 54*(2), 74–84.

Fawcett, J. (2005). Criteria for evaluation of theory. *Nursing Science Quarterly, 18*(2), 131–135.

Filatotchev, I., & Nakajma, C. (2014). Corporate governance, responsible managerial behavior, and corporate social responsibility: Organizational efficiency versus organizational legitimacy. *Academy of Management Perspectives, 1*(28), 289–306.

Froman, L. (2010). Positive psychology in the workplace. *Journal of Adult Development, 17*(2), 59–69.

Goldsmith, M. (2010). Sharing leadership to maximize talent. *Harvard Business Review*. Retrieved February 5, 2015, from https://hbr.org/2010/05/sharing-leadership-to-maximize/

Institute of Medicine (IOM) Committee on Quality of Health Care in America. (2001). *Crossing the quality chasm: A new health system for the 21st century*. Washington, DC: National Academies Press.

Kaner, S. (2014). *Facilitators guide to participatory decision-making* (2nd ed.). San Francisco, CA: John Wiley & Sons.

Laschinger, H. K. S., & Fida, R. (2014). New nurses burnout and workplace well-being: The influence of authentic leadership and psychological capital. *Burnout Research, 1*(1), 19–28.

Lefton, C. (2012). Strengthening the workforce through meaningful recognition. *Nursing Economic$, 30*(6), 331–338.

Lewis, M., & Pettersson, G. (2009). *Governance in health care delivery: Raising performance* (World Bank Working Paper #5074). Washington, DC: World Bank. Retrieved February 5, 2015, from http://www.g8.utoronto.ca/conferences/2010/ghdp/lewis-pettersson.pdf

Llewellyn, A., & Leonard, M. (2009). *Nursing case management review and resource manual* (3rd ed.). Silver Spring, MD: American Nurses Credentialing Center.

Lovan, R. W., Shaffer, R., & Murray, M. (Eds.). (2004). *Participatory governance: Planning, conflict mediation and public-decision making in civil society*. London, UK: Ashgate Publishing.

Lowell General Hospital. (2015a). *Mission statement*. Retrieved from http://www.lowellgeneral.org/about-lgh/our-mission

Lowell General Hospital. (2015b). *Nursing philosophy*. Retrieved from http://www .lowellgeneral.org/search?q=nursing+philosophy

Luthans, F., & Youssef, C. M. (2004). Human, social, and now positive psychological capital management. *Organizational Dynamics, 33*, 143–160

Luthans, F., Avey, J. B., Avolio, B. J., & Peterson, S. J. (2010). The development and resulting performance impact of positive psychological capital. *Human Resource Development Quarterly, 21*(1), 41–66.

Marquis, B. L., & Huston, C. J. (2000). *Leadership roles and management functions in nursing theory and application*. Philadelphia, PA: Lippincott, Williams, and Wilkins.

Maslow, A. H. (1943). A theory of human motivation. *Psychology Review, 50*(4), 370–396.

Maslow, A. H. (1954). *Motivation and personality*. New York, NY: Harper.

McHugh, M. D., Berez, J., & Small, D. S. (2013). Hospitals with higher nurse staffing had lower odds of readmissions penalties than hospitals with lower staffing. *Health Affairs, 32*(10), 1740–1747.

Mensik, J. S., Martin, D. M., Scott, K. A., & Horton, K. (2011). Development of a professional nursing framework: The journey toward nursing excellence. *Journal of Nursing Administration, 41*(6), 259–264.

Meyers, M., & Costanzo, C. (2015). Shared governance in a clinic system. *Nursing Administration Quarterly, 39*(1), 51–57.

Misra, S., Allison, M., & Perry, E. (2014). Doing more with more: Putting shared leadership into practice. *Nonprofit Quarterly*. Retrieved from https://nonprofitquarterly.org/management/24051-doing-more-with-more-putting-shared-leadership-into-practice.html

Needleman, J., Buerhaus, P., Mattke, S., Stewart, M., & Zelevinsky, K. (2002). Nurse-staffing levels and the quality of care in hospitals. *New England Journal of Medicine, 346*(22), 1715–1722.

Nelson, B., & Spitzer, D. (2003). *The 1001 rewards and recognition fieldbook*. New York, NY: Workman Publishing.

O'Grady, T. P. (1987). Shared governance and new organizational models. *Nursing Economic$, 5*(6), 281–286.

O'Grady, T. P. (2001). Is shared governance still relevant? *Journal of Nursing Administration, 31*(10), 468–473.

Owens, A. L., & Cleaves, J. (2012). Then and now: Updating clinical nurse advancement programs. *Nursing, 42*(10), 15–17.

Pearce, C. L., & Conger, J. A. (2003). *Shared leadership: Reframing the hows and whys of leadership*. Thousand Oaks, CA: Sage.

Rafferty, A. M., Clarke, S. P., Coles, J., Ball, J., James, P., McKee, M., & Aiken, L. H. (2007). Outcomes of variation in hospital nurse staffing in English hospitals: Cross-sectional analysis of survey data and discharge records. *International Journal of Nursing Studies, 44*(2), 175–182.

Ravari, A., Bazargan-Hejazi, S., Ebadi, A., Mirzaei, T., & Oshvandi, K. (2013). Work values and job satisfaction: A qualitative study of Iranian Nurses. *Nursing Ethics, 20*(4), 448–458.

Riley, J., Rolband, D. H., James, D., & Norton, H. J. (2009). Clinical ladder: Nurses' perceptions and satisfiers. *Journal of Nursing Administration, 39*(4), 182–188.

Riordan, C. M. (2013, April). Foster a culture of gratitude. *Harvard Business Review,* p. 40. Retrieved from https://hbr.org/2013/04/foster-a-culture-of-gratitude

Sally, D. (2002). Co-leadership: Lessons from republican Rome. *California Business Review, 44*(1), 84–99.

Scholle, S. H., Torda, P., Peikes, D., Han, E., & Genevro, J. (2010). *Engaging patients in the medical home* (AHRQ Publication No. 10-0083-EF). Rockville, MD: Agency for Healthcare Research and Quality.

Serratt, T., Meyer, S., & Chapman, S. A. (2014). Enforcement of hospital nurse staffing regulations across the United States: Progress or stalemate? *Policy and Politics in Nursing Practice, 15*(1–2), 21–29.

Smith, M. C., & Parker, M. E. (2015). *Nursing theories and nursing practice* (4th ed.). Philadelphia, PA: F. A. Davis.

Snellman, I., & Gedda, K. M. (2012). The value ground of nursing. *Nursing Ethics, 19*(6), 714–726.

Tourangeau, A. E., Cranley, L. A., & Jeffs, L. (2006). Impact of nursing on patient mortality: A review and related policy implications. *Quality and Safety in Health Care, 15*(1), 4–6.

Tourangeau, A. E., Doran, D. M., McGillis Hall, L., O'Brien Pallas, L., Pringle, D., Tu, J. V., & Cranley, L. A. (2007). Impact of hospital nursing care on 30-day mortality for acute medical patients. *Journal of Advanced Nursing, 57*(1), 32–44.

Watson, J. (2006). Caring theory as an ethical guide to administrative and clinical practices. *Nursing Administration Quarterly, 30*(1), 48–55.

Watson, J. (2012). *Caring science: A theory of nursing.* Sudbury, MA: Jones & Bartlett.

Winslow, S. A., Fickley, S., Knight, D., Richards, K., Rosson, J., & Rumbley, N. (2011). Staff nurses revitalize a clinical ladder program through shared governance. *Journal for Nurses in Staff Development, 27*(1), 13–17.

CHAPTER 5

Application of Professional Practice Models: Implementation

Implementation plan, implementation strategies

By the end of this chapter, readers will be able to:

1. Describe the components of a professional practice model (PPM) implementation plan
2. Recognize the difference between goals and objectives
3. State measurable goals
4. Choose implementation strategies that align with nursing values and organizational strengths
5. Enrich the implementation plan by including encouraging behaviors and reinforcement techniques

THE IMPLEMENTATION PLAN

Once the "thinking" work of designing a professional practice model (PPM) has been completed, it is appropriate to begin acting. In this case, action refers to initiating the phases of integration (see Figure 2.1) by defining the work that is to be done (planning), designing evidence-based strategies (generating), and assigning appropriate responsibilities and time frames for completion (accountability). In this chapter, focus will be placed on implementing the application phase. Although this sounds like a simple task, implementation

plans frequently fail "not because the new strategies or goals are inappropriate but rather because organizations are unable to successfully implement
them" (Caldwell, Chatman, O'Reilly, Ormiston, & Lapiz, 2008, p. 125).

> Integrating a professional practice model (PPM) is not simply a function of
> drawing a diagram, adopting a theory, providing some education, or reorganizing
> units. Successful integration requires that leaders, employees, and work groups
> modify the way they do things. In fact, integrating a model is a major culture
> change that necessitates new behaviors and revised ways of thinking.

PLANNING

When approached with discipline and full participation, planning, generating, and establishing accountability for implementation involves the following: establishing a committee; emphasizing the certainty of the PPM; reflecting
on the position of the organization relative to the PPM; setting strategic goals;
creating action-oriented objectives (in measurable terms); selecting evidence-
based implementation strategies to meet specific objectives; building in ongoing support and enrichment activities; prioritizing strategies; and assigning
responsibility and expectations for completion (Figure 5.1).

Step 1 includes establishing a diverse committee that includes representatives from all nursing levels. The membership of the implementation committee should include key nursing staff leaders (e.g., the chairs of nursing
councils, especially the practice council) in order to take advantage of their
experience and expertise and enlist their help in implementing the plans they
helped shape. For example, those champions of the PPM (e.g., those who best
defended its concepts and advocated for its adoption) would be ideal committee members. In addition, the committee should comprise selected members of
nursing administration, nursing education, advanced practitioners, and others
who can offer important insights and support to this group. The final implementation committee membership ideally should be around eight to 15 members (depending on the size of the health system).

The implementation committee elects a leader or facilitator, establishes
a routine meeting schedule with rules regarding participation and processes,
and forms communication and feedback processes. Developing a realistic
timeline for completion of a PPM implementation plan and sticking to it will
expedite the committee's progress. Keeping the focus on those forces impacting future nursing practice as well as incorporating best evidence into the
implementation will inform the quality of the result.

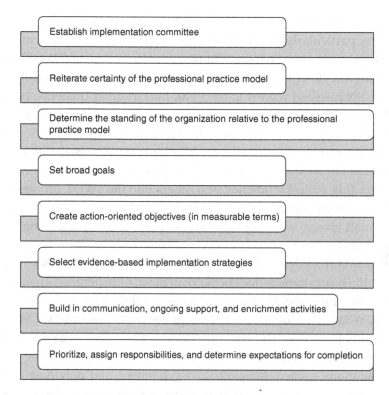

Figure 5.1 Implementation process.

Step 2 involves committee members' strong and continuing support of those convictions that formed the basis for the newly designed PPM, being careful to tie the model to the organizational mission and nursing values statements. Feedback from patients and families and administration concerning the value of the model extends its validity, strengthening buy-in. Such endorsement reinforces the shared vision for nursing practice, ensures that the beliefs and values of nursing are respected and upheld, and helps commit resources to the integration process.

Although it is important that the professional practice model is consistently described and appreciated by all nurses, other health professionals, senior administrators, and even the board of directors, it is especially crucial that key nursing leaders understand and embrace the model. It will provide important defining parameters for them as they develop, assume accountability for, and support implementation of the plan. Consistency of mind-set among the key nursing leaders regarding the professional practice of nursing as it is situated in the organization offers a strong platform from which to actualize the implementation process and optimize successful integration.

Step 3 involves reflecting back on the internal organizational readiness evidence, particularly the gap analysis (see Chapter 2), and completing a quick strengths, weaknesses, and opportunities/threats (SWOT) analysis (Andrews, 1971) to identify the relative position of the organization (specifically nursing) related to the PPM, the customer (patients, families, health care providers, suppliers, the community, others), the discipline, and other competitors. Involving diverse points of view in the SWOT analysis expands perspectives, thereby improving the possibility of gaining enough knowledge of current nursing practice and its effectiveness. In fact, including patients, families, and others into the SWOT process leverages the analysis even further. Individuals on the implementation committee or small groups working together can participate in collecting SWOT information.

In a SWOT analysis, strengths refer to those nursing attributes or activities that the health system does better than most, or better than anyone else, in the competitive area. Pertinent responses are elicited by asking questions, such as, What do we do well (vis-à-vis professional practice)? Or, What do we do better than most? Reflecting on aspects of practice—such as quality of services; resources spent; application of skills, including technology, innovative solutions applied, professional development, and providing optimal patient experiences—allows for more in-depth analysis. Following are some examples of nursing strengths:

- Lower rates of adverse outcomes (medication errors, pressure ulcers, falls)
- Higher percentages of nurses with certification
- Greater percentages of patients who rate the patient experience higher (compared to similar institutions)
- RNs with proficiency in specific technologies
- Higher-than-average nurse retention rates

Weaknesses include those attributes and activities that, if substantially improved, would provide nursing with additional probabilities for success. Receiving multiple views from key nurses; leaders within the organization; as well as patients, families, and those outside the organization, ensures that all key weaknesses are identified. Pertinent questions to ask include What do we do not so well (vis-à-vis professional practice)? What should be improved? Are there mistakes we need to avoid? Do others (both within and outside the system) see nursing weaknesses as we do, or differently? Honest and realistic evaluation of nursing practice is essential. Following are some examples of nursing practice weaknesses:

- A higher percentage of RNs without recent continuing education
- Little or no use of evidence in practice
- Higher or lower rates of nursing hours per patient day (relative to similar organizations)
- Less-than-average RN engagement
- Poorer patient outcomes

Opportunities are often the product of trends or conditions appearing outside of the organization but within nursing. Some examples are consolidation of services (such as merging inpatient and outpatient services for a population), acquisition of additional health systems, translating new evidence into practice (e.g., transition programs), innovative clinical advancement systems, novel ways of staffing or use of resources, or authentic educational resources (e.g., a university close by).

> Recognizing the development of trends or future changes comes from effective networking, reading the literature, being aware of the "competition," benchmarking, and scanning the environment, all important functions of leadership.

Following are examples of nursing opportunities:

- A formalized academic–service partnership
- Forward-thinking onboarding strategies for nurse leaders
- Active use of new evidence (e.g., oral care practices)
- Focused sabbaticals for selected nursing staff

Threats are the obstacles nursing faces or will face in trying to implement the newly developed PPM. Threats may include lack of resources, poor leadership, negative views of nursing's role in the system, and lack of needed technology.

> Recognition of real or perceived threats is important in the development of implementation strategies and critical to avoiding surprises that hinder goal achievement.

Following are some examples of threats:

- Majority of nursing leadership staff is maturing (retirements looming) and no succession plan has been created.

- Local competition is strong.
- Changes in reimbursement mechanisms are on the horizon.
- Patient volume is fading in areas of nursing core competency.

A thorough SWOT analysis, with full participation of all members of the implementation committee and across key constituencies, sets up the foundation for informed implementation approaches.

The next step includes thorough goal setting, beginning with a series of statements that describe the desired nursing practice in a specified number of years (e.g., 3, 5, 10 years from the present). The length of time to the desired nursing practice is determined by the implementation committee.

It is important that a series of significant goals regarding organizational professional nursing practice, preferably in the form of status statements describing the preferred practice of nursing, be developed.

Goals are broad targets or intentions that are proposed to describe the desired end state—in this case, the fully integrated PPM. Setting goals inspires success and provides documentation for celebrating accomplishments. As such they should be agreed on and be significant even beyond the specific health system. Goals might cover a variety of categories, and are then stated as follows (in declarative statements):

- Professional nursing practice at _____ will respond to the needs and preferences of patients and families.
- Professional nurses at _____ will be knowledgeable of, possess the skills for, and value the PPM.
- Employees at all levels throughout the system will be aware of, accept, and support the PPM as the basis for nursing practice.
- Adequate resources will be allocated for PPM integration.
- Professional nurses at _____ will be fairly represented on internal shared governance committees, key hospital-wide committees, and at least three external community or professional organizations.

Once broad goals have been specified, the implementation committee might look back at the SWOT results and recommend modifications of the goals (based on available strengths or to augment noted weaknesses). This might mean identifying potential new goals or suggesting changes in emphasis in order to pave the way for the more specific objective setting.

Developing objectives that relate to each goal requires recognition of the distinction between goals and objectives.

> Whereas goals are broad and affirm the desired end state, objectives are specific, measurable, and occur in the shorter term. They include those specific actions that will be used to direct activities required to meet the established goals. Objectives provide the level of specificity necessary to evaluate goal attainment. Stating them correctly is crucial since they will later function as success criteria and provide the basis for regular feedback.

Using the SMART language as an example, objectives should be specific, measurable, achievable, realistic, and timely (Doran, 1981). Specificity refers to understanding (i.e., clear and free of jargon); the terms used are well defined, the actions are focused, and there is enough detail that those involved know what to do. Avoiding words that have vague meanings and using action verbs, such as *design, develop, build*, and *conduct*, assists in knowing *what* to do. Naming those involved (*who*), including *when* the activity is to be completed and addressing *how* exactly the action will be completed, is important. Finally each objective should be neatly aligned with a goal or goals and then again with the overarching PPM. This answers the question, "*Why* is it important to do this?

> Setting objectives that are measurable (quantifiable) will later provide tangible evidence of their attainment (specific behaviors that can be observed or the amount of change expected) and is crucial for the evaluation plan (Chapter 6) as well as organizational documentation of the evaluation plan's investment in the professional practice model.

Measurable objectives provide a reference point from which changes in goals can be clearly measured. Asking the questions: How will I know when this objective has been achieved? Are there any existing measurements (questionnaires, observations) that I can use to evaluate its completion? and What milestones can I use to track progress toward completion that will ensure a quality objective? It is impossible to determine whether objectives have been met unless they can be measured; thus it is crucial to perform this task correctly. Writing objectives this way does not come easy and takes experience—consulting with an educator or researcher may be helpful.

In the SMART example, *achievable* is linked to *measurable*, but refers more to the practicality of attainment. If others have done something successfully, or if members of the planning team have positive experiences with an objective, then it is more likely to be successful. Realistic objectives are those that can be achieved with the available resources (skills, funding, equipment, time, staff) or at least there is a reasonable chance of meeting them. Finally, timing of objectives, particularly identifying the point in time that attainment is expected, enables efficiency of implementation. Example objectives written in response to a set goal are listed as follows:

- *Goal*: Employees at all levels throughout the system will be aware of, accept, and support the PPM as the basis for nursing practice.
- *Objective 1:* By May 2017, at least 90% of employees in each department will sign an agreement to uphold the PPM.
- *Objective 2:* By October 2017, at least 90% of employees in each department can state three components of the PPM.
- *Objective 3:* By November 2017, at least 90% of employees in each department can verbally defend the PPM as the basis for nursing practice.

> For each goal, there are an infinite number of objectives that can be developed. It is wise to include only those that are necessary, are realistic and measurable, and, most important, are relevant to the professional practice model.

Building in objectives for monitoring and modifying strategies based on changes in the external environment or the organization is crucial. For example, objectives for taking advantage of unexpected changes, such as more engaged or new top leadership, reductions in dedicated resources, or changes in patient or staff characteristics, should be anticipated and designed into the implementation process. From the specific objectives, the committee can proceed to select those specific strategies that will be used to meet the objectives and overall goals.

IMPLEMENTATION STRATEGIES

Changing behaviors and ways of thinking on a systematic level requires varied evidence-based strategies such as learning opportunities, the alignment of roles and responsibilities, reinforcement activities, redesigning workflow (if necessary), effective communication, and ongoing support and advancement strategies. There is no one set of strategies that fits a particular health system. Rather, based on the initial readiness assessment, SWOT analysis, the stated objectives and PPM itself, organizational priorities, and the evidence base, a set of strategies is selected that best fits the health systems and its employees. After initial development of selected strategies, a review of the implementation goals and objectives may require the implementation committee to recommend alternative approaches or methods to achieve the stated objectives. To begin Step 6, ask questions from the perspective of the patient/family such as:

- What are the needs and processes of patients/families?
- What is it that nursing can do (as defined by the PPM) to increase value as perceived by the patient/family?
- What factors are important in the patient/family decision-making process?
- How can patient-family engagement be improved?

Or, ask from the perspective of the discipline of nursing:

- What are the best practices of others in terms of improving nursing practice using a PPM?
- What is known (through an appraisal of current evidence) about effective integration of PPMs?
- What do professional organizations report related to excellence in nursing practice?

A disciplined approach should be undertaken to answer these questions and identify those strategies that are evidence based and will lead to successful results (effectiveness) while preserving efficiency. For example, to address learning needs of employees, a face-to-face classroom approach as well as several online modular methods or a combination strategy as suggested by best evidence may be recommended. Based on the unique organization (personnel, resources, etc.) and the needs of its employees for integrating a PPM, decisions can be made using several different approaches (e.g., group consensus, democratic voting). Whatever the specific approach applied, specific criteria for evaluating and choosing among many possible strategies should be agreed on (see Table 5.1). Based on these or other agreed-upon criteria, strategies can be evaluated, chosen, re-evaluated, and finally selected for implementation.

Some systems prefer to engage consultants with expertise in PPM implementation to assist with strategy formulation and integration procedures. Others do it alone. Regardless of the approach, it is crucial to consider

Table 5.1 Criteria for Selecting Implementation Strategies

- Value—Will the strategy contribute to meeting agreed-upon goals?

- Appropriateness—Is the strategy consistent with the organization's mission, nursing values, and PPM?

- Feasibility—Is the strategy practical, given personnel and financial resources and system capacity?

- Acceptability—Is the strategy acceptable to the key staff, and other stakeholders?

- Cost–benefit—Is the strategy likely to lead to sufficient benefits to justify the costs in time and other resources?

- Timing—Can and should the organization implement this strategy at this time, given external factors and competing demands?

multiple evidence-based options and use those experts with considerable experience in implementing new programs. Choosing strategies involves careful consideration of who in the organization (or resources outside the organization that are made available) have the expertise to successfully implement the action. For example, if an implementation goal is to deliver care consistent with a specific nursing theory, then a key strategy might be to increase knowledge of the theory or to revise current job descriptions to support consistency between nursing actions and the theory. After acquiring knowledge of the theory or seeking guidance on nursing job descriptions through reading the literature and/or consultation with the theorist, specified individuals within the organization may take on the responsibility for implementing this strategy.

> Choosing which actions to use in a specific context requires achieving a balance between fidelity to the implementation goals (and overarching professional practice model) and the criteria, as well as accommodating local needs, including differences among departments in a health system.

Some (but certainly not all) strategies that might be used when implementing a PPM are discussed in the following sections.

Education

Data indicate that providing education and training to individual health care personnel is not enough to change practice. In particular, didactic education used alone has been shown to be less effective than interactive learning opportunities (Bluestone et al., 2013). Yet, many who implement new PPMs develop traditional instructional programs as the *only* means to change behavior. Some of these are as little as one 2-hour classroom session.

To begin, it is helpful to assess the educational levels and best learning techniques of current employees. Using this information, designing an experiential approach to education, using effective interactive learning techniques, such as case studies, games, point-of-care learning (e.g., clinical rounds), problem-based learning activities, role playing, peer learning, focused assignments, group simulations, and others, is more useful than the passive transfer of information used in traditional classrooms. For example, from a case study used to set up a clinical situation, learners could use the selected nursing theory to develop the plan of care. Or, using another clinical situation, learners could assume roles (assigned by the educator) to perform their respective duties according to a revised nursing job description. These forms of learning tend to "stick" with learners and address both the cognitive and psychomotor requirements of learning. To effectively attend to the affective learning dimension, helping learners perceive the patient's view is crucial. For example, listening to patient stories, patient participation in the classroom, individual written and group reflections, and working through ethical dilemmas help to instill values and attitudes that are aligned with the chosen PPM.

> Such an active and reflective instructional approach addresses many different learning styles and allows students (in this case, staff RNs) to become engaged both in and outside the classroom, to receive immediate feedback, create a personal connection to the content, practice important skills, build self-esteem, reflect on the course content, accept responsibility for learning, and see the value of each learning experience in terms of how it informs practice.

Most important, research consistently supports that students learn better when they are engaged in the process (Meeks, Heit, & Page, 2009).

Within the context of experiential learning activities, it is also useful to present data about the underlying theoretical portion of the PPM in terms of its benefits to improving quality of care, its relationship to RN work satisfaction, and how others have incorporated it. Such evidence provides nurses with important reference points from which to base their evolving practice. Having participants appraise themselves, review pertinent literature, and relay their findings to others is a useful experiential learning approach for practicing clinicians.

Experiential learning starts with the educator. It is vital that clinical educators establish an excitement for learning, embody the professional practice model, and create opportunities for active student participation. Teaching strategies must be carefully selected to support student engagement both on and off the clinical unit, and be reflective enough to allow deep contemplation about the content. Finally, reinforcing activities (particularly those that occur in the clinical area) keep the content alive, allow for updates, and strengthen the underpinning professional practice model.

Modifying Work Roles and Responsibilities

As the PPM becomes more understood in the organization, it follows that some work-role revisions might be necessary. These revisions most often include RN roles, but also frequently include those that support RN work (e.g., unlicensed assistive personnel) and those that complement nursing work (e.g., other health care providers).

With respect to the chosen professional practice model, clear roles help employees understand their specific duties and responsibilities, the importance of their obligations, and their overall position with respect to the organizational mission and specified nursing values.

For nursing, clear work roles contribute to overall quality by identifying the most appropriate personnel for the revised clinical functions and ensure that the work carried out is aligned with the PPM.

Conducting a role-delineation (or job analysis) review helps to fully understand and describe the current duties and responsibilities of a position as well as the knowledge, skills, and abilities required to perform well in the position. The aim is to have a complete picture of the position—*what* is actually done and *how*—in relation to the PPM. More specifically, describing practice expectations and performance requirements as they link to the underlying theoretical framework of the PPM provides the necessary background for deciding to revise existing job descriptions. Because this is the basis of most human resource activities, it is prudent to involve this department in the process.

Role delineation usually involves collecting information about the responsibilities associated with the current roles, identifying knowledge domains and required skills, analyzing and interpreting the results, creating revised job descriptions (if necessary), confirming the link between revised performance expectations, knowledge, and skills and the underlying nursing theoretical framework, and developing a final detailed performance description.

The types of information collected during role delineation are specific to each organization; however, typical kinds of information that are gathered include (Roberts & Hughes, 2013):

- Details of most common duties
- Supervisory responsibilities
- Educational requirements
- Other special qualifications
- Experience required
- Equipment/tools used
- Frequency of supervision
- Relationships with others in the organization
- Authority for decision making
- Responsibility for records/reports/files
- Working conditions
- Physical demands of the job
- Mental demands of the job

Information about employee roles can be gathered using qualitative or quantitative techniques such as interviews, questionnaires, observations, and activity logs. Using a sampling plan for gathering information helps identify those who are experts in the specific role and facilitates efficiency. Deciding on the instruments—qualitative or quantitative or both—including the validity of the particular tools used, as well as selecting the data-collecting methods, safeguards credibility of results.

Interpreting the results through task summaries, priority ratings, or other qualitative techniques may require an experienced evaluator/researcher or consultation with a statistician. Validating the results is crucial; soliciting feedback from those already in the role facilitates "buy-in" with regard to any revisions. Conducting a series of meetings with groups of interested employees, leaders, and human resource personnel allows for full participation. Using a nonleader facilitator to focus and advance the process along is helpful. Such a process gives voice to the employee and allows for creativity in any revisions. Benchmarking the results with others who use a similar PPM validates any revisions.

With this information in hand, a thorough evaluation of those categories of employees who will be delivering care according to the specified PPM can be gleaned.

> Although revision of job descriptions is not required, oftentimes it is necessary to ensure the accurate delivery of services according to the specified model. Specifying job performance expectations must appropriately reflect the responsibilities of all groups of employees who will participate in the delivery of care according to the professional practice model.

Setting decision rules or criteria to retain or remove certain tasks is helpful in this process. For example, a retained task must be significant to the practice (as defined by the PPM and the amount of time spent performing it), whereas one that is removed may be less significant with less percentages of time spent performing it.

Confirming the link between retained responsibilities, knowledge domains, skills, and the nursing theoretical underpinnings of the PPM is crucial. Using a chart or crosswalk approach may facilitate this process (Table 5.2). The leader plays an important role in providing feedback to employees about expected work behaviors and can also motivate employees to participate in the process by allowing them to converse openly and safely about the work. Leaders, consultants, and others who are experts in the PPM can offer suggestions concerning the alignment of nursing work with nursing values.

Finally, using the results of the information gathered, revised job descriptions that are well aligned with the PPM can be developed.

Table 5.2 Example Link Between Theoretical Underpinnings, Associated Knowledge and Skills, and Retained Nursing Responsibilities

Theoretical Underpinnings	Knowledge and Skills	Retained Responsibilities
Quality-Caring Model[©]: Relational nature of human beings	The "whole" person, interdependence with others, four essential relationships	Holistic nursing assessment, collaborative relationships with the health care team, caring for self and the community served
Caring relationships	Caring factors	Initiating, cultivating, and sustaining caring relationships

A well-written job description creates the basis for employee selection, hiring, performance management, and advancement. Thus, the job description is a critical document that is often overlooked in the enthusiasm of integrating a professional practice model. Clarifying what nurses and those who support them do facilitates the accurate delivery of professionally inspired nursing practice and provides an opportunity to focus on meaningful work that enhances patient outcomes.

Redesigning Clinical Workflow

Clinical workflow details sequentially how clinical work actually gets done; it comprises the actual steps performed by various staff members for a certain process (Brixey, Robinson, Turley, & Zhang, 2010). For example, during admission to an acute-care hospital, the patient and family enter the unit; a history and physical assessment are completed and documented accordingly; orders are received, processed, and charged; a care plan is begun; responsibilities are assigned; and, one hopes, the discharge process is initiated.

This one process alone duplicates the services of multiple workers rendering it a communication nightmare that is somewhat inefficient, but most important, it may not be organized around the patient or in accordance with the underlying nursing values that determined the PPM. Or, take the case of medication administration. This is a complex process in most health systems involving any numbers of medications and patients, multiple departments, policies and procedures, procurement and safe administration, environmental concerns, preparation time, documentation, gathering equipment and supplies, and so on. As with the example of the admission process, duplication of work, adequate communication, and expert professional practice delivered in harmony with the PPM may be in jeopardy.

Although clinical workflow related to electronic health record implementation has been recently assessed and reported (Bowens, Frye, & Jones, 2010; Campion, Johnson, Paxton, Mushlin, & Sedrakyan, 2014), little has been reported with respect to PPM integration. Therefore, when integrating a PPM, assessing and adjusting clinical workflow in order to ensure that professional nurses are performing in accord with the model is essential. Clinical workflow impacts care delivery in terms of its safety and quality, efficiency, information transfer, coordination of services, and interactions (in terms of holistically meeting patient/family needs). In the acute care environment, nurses have traditionally spent a good portion of their time (greater than 50%) in indirect patient care (Hendricks & Baume, 2008; Upenieks, Akhavan, & Kotlerman, 2008). The Transforming Care at the Bedside (TCAB) initiative recently began to transform work processes for maximum value. In this demonstration project, front-line nurses were engaged to advance safety and consistency of care, promote enthusiasm for the work, increase patient and family satisfaction, encourage innovation, and add value (Dearmon et al., 2013). Direct care and value-added care times increased each year of the project (above the national median), overtime decreased, and falls-with-harm rates significantly decreased on TCAB units compared to non-TCAB units (Dearmon et al., 2013). Although limitations were noted in this project, it provides interesting information regarding how nursing work can be redesigned to meet established goals.

Redesigning clinical workflow in accord with the chosen PPM involves a commitment to the model's underlying guiding values, support for those measurable objectives developed in the plan, and collaboration among a number of employees and the human resources department. Although it is also not necessary to modify clinical workflow, it is important to consider this workflow when implementing a PPM.

Some organizations use a workflow map to document and diagram important unit-based clinical processes, and then critically analyze their effectiveness and efficiency, particularly in the eyes of the customer (patients and families). Analysis should note instances in which there are duplications of services, multiple steps involved, and whether the needs of customers are met with the current process. Next, areas in need of improvement are identified, and decisions with regard to whether current processes should be modified are made.

> If clinical workflow modification is deemed necessary, considering how patient and family needs could be best met, identifying whose expertise would best actualize the professional practice model in a given process, whether the number of steps could be reduced or combined, and then remodeling the process to optimize adherence to the professional practice model is a good approach to take in the modification process.

Enlisting the support of patients and families, staff members, leadership, other providers, and external consultants facilitates clinical workflow redesign while empowering clinicians in the process. Oftentimes, this process evolves into a revised patient care delivery system (see Chapter 4) that will better define nursing roles and responsibilities, enhance communication, ensure resources and assignments remain true to the PPM, and provide the basis for environmental supports.

Effective Communication

Communication is a critical implementation strategy. During any type of change, including integrating a new PPM, uncertainty about "what it means to me" often leads to job insecurity, which can translate into feelings of anxiety, unrest, doubt, and lack of confidence in the leadership. Communication is a two-way process of reaching mutual understanding, in which participants not only exchange (encode–decode) information, news, ideas, and feelings, but also create and share meaning ("Communication," 2015). It involves conveying messages or information accurately and in enough detail to generate clarity and trust in the sender. It should also incorporate a reasonable delivery method and connect with the beliefs of the receiver. Much evidence exists about the importance of good communication during change processes (Saruhan, 2014). Specifying the actual communication strategies will strengthen their success and alert the leadership to their important role. Communicating consistently and frequently, using multiple channels and mechanisms as soon as new information is available, and including the rationale for new behaviors that align with the chosen PPM is paramount. Conveying transparency of the process (including the delivery of "bad news") instills trust, a factor that enables successful integration projects (Schlicter & Rose, 2013). Of course, providing opportunities for asking questions, clarifying information, providing input, and soliciting alternative ideas is a part of the communication process that leaders often miss. In fact, face-to-face, two-way communication is most beneficial. Tailoring messages to the receiver is also important because it alleviates concerns and fears (such as, Why are we doing this? Is the health system in trouble? Am I still relevant? How much will my job change?). Often, formal communication channels are considered the only source of information when planning a large system change, but the informal channel (aka the grapevine) can be a source of important information, *if* used effectively by leadership.

Because information needs are usually determined by the individual, any time there is a void (as perceived by employees) it tends to be filled with something. In health systems, gossip, rumors, exaggerations, resistance, and even outright sabotage can ensue when employees perceive lack of communication. These behaviors pose risks to the implementation of a PPM because they distract employees from their existing roles and responsibilities and limit their contribution to building the new model. Thus, communicating proactively, obtaining feedback often, and recognizing the growing impact of social networking on the grapevine are important leadership strategies. Finally, continuing effective communication strategies throughout the implementation period (which is extensive, often spanning years) is a challenge but is necessary.

Ongoing Support and Enrichment

Encouragement and reinforcement are required to sustain engagement in the implementation process as well as to alter behaviors. Being encouraging involves verbal and nonverbal messages that are reassuring, positive, enthusiastic, and the source of ongoing inspiration. It assumes that individuals are intrinsically motivated and allows room for expression of feelings (both good and bad; Duffy, 2009).

> A supportive tone maintains a sense of ease with the process, sustains faith in the professional practice model, and empowers others—it is a leadership responsibility.

Reinforcement is a consequence of behaviors (Skinner, 1974) that, when used positively, emphasizes important details, thereby enhancing learning and strengthening desirable behaviors. Leaders who use positive reinforcement must first recognize those behaviors they want repeated (which requires some pre-planning), and then, using strong motivators (reinforcements) and proper timing, offer the stimulus. Leaders who are encouraging and who use reinforcing techniques build a foundation of trust that allows for feelings of security, dependability, and confidence in the process.

Creating Safe Space

Safe space is an environmental and relational characteristic in which one feels relaxed, comfortable, and can express oneself fully without fear of reprisals (in the form of feeling uncomfortable in any way, judged, or disrespected). It is an authentic environment where diverse workers feel they each matter and their individual contribution facilitates system progress. Safe space enables new ways of thinking, creativity, and risk taking (Llerena-Quinn, 2013).

Leaders generate "safe space" when input is acknowledged and appreciated, when opportunities for meaningful inclusion are presented, behaviors are open and flexible (e.g., transparent), the atmosphere is calm, and communication tends to be positive.

Using open-ended questions that reflect listening techniques, strategies, such as appreciative inquiry (Lamont, 2013), ongoing monitoring of participants' comfort levels, self-awareness, and summaries of what is said during communications, leaders can impart a feeling of security, open dialogue, and inclusivity, which is necessary for easing the transition to new ways of practicing. In essence, practicing authentic leadership (George, 2004)—leading from the inside out—enhances health systems' capacity to embrace emerging views, working together versus working separately, and gives voice to those gaps in patient care that might be reduced by the PPM. Leaders' responses during this process provide the guidance needed to attain successful integration.

Coaching

Coaching is the art of guiding another person, persons, or human systems toward a fulfilling future (Hudson, 1999, p. 22). Another definition is "partnering with others in a thought-provoking and creative process that inspires them to maximize their personal and professional potential" (International Coach Federation, 2015, p. 1). Coaching focuses on the client or, in this case the employee, and uses a customized approach that best fits his or her needs. Coaching is an individually tailored method of development that empowers others to ultimately take responsibility for themselves through making necessary changes in their professional and personal lives (Cummings & Worley, 2015). It involves relationships, nurturing, teaching, supporting, and listening. Providing coaching resources to nurses often facilitates the development of new behaviors.

Providing Feedback

Feedback (2015) is a response to, a reaction, or an assessment of another. In the workplace, it usually occurs in relation to performance and is intended to enhance learning or guide performance. Yet, some employees only receive feedback during the formal, annual evaluation process. Anseel and Lievens (2007) showed that evaluative feedback did not improve employee motivation and satisfaction, but rather that employees welcomed more supportive,

developmental feedback. Other research supports that supervisor developmental feedback is positively associated with positive employee work attitudes and behavior (Joo & Park, 2010).

Developmental feedback is defined as the extent to which supervisors
provide information that enables employees to learn, develop, and improve
at work (Zhou, 2003).

Especially during a period of transition (such as integrating a professional
practice model), giving and receiving feedback is crucial. Employees closest
to the bedside often have a good understanding of day-to-day operations and
know those small details that impact quality patient care. Providing meaningful
feedback to them less formally and more frequently raises awareness and
provides more direction in terms of next steps.

Using informal conversations or short notes personalizes the message,
encourages two-way communication, and lessens the feedback cycle. Occasionally, providing feedback to an entire team, especially if data can back
up their performance, is valuable. This encourages collaboration and cele-
brates working together. When clinicians are actually making progress (e.g.,
a new milestone has been reached) making a big deal about it provides an
opportunity to drive even more positive changes in behavior and reinstill
those nursing values into the implementation process. Effective feedback
provides actionable insight to employees, empowering them to own their
progress and, ultimately, drive integration of the PPM. Although feedback is
generally considered good, there are emotional aspects of feedback that warrant attention. In fact, emotional reactions resulting from feedback mediate
the relationship between feedback and counterproductive behavior, turnover
intentions, citizenship, and affective commitment (Belschak & Den Hartog,
2009). From their studies, Belschak and Den Hartog (2009) imply that negative feedback, especially when given publically, may drive undesired attitudes and behaviors. Furthermore, Nowack (2014) indicates that negative
feedback produces physiologic effects as well in terms of eliciting the stress
response and provoking inflammation, depression, and fatigue. Thus, providing feedback that considers the intended receiver in a clear, constructive,
and supportive manner may be less emotionally charged.

Feedback focused on behaviors that receivers can do something about, rather
than on individuals themselves, that is given in the spirit of helping is most
developmental.

In fact, the amount of information given should reflect the recipient's needs. Overloading on feedback reduces the receiver's ability to effectively use it and, more often than not, when leaders give more feedback than can be used, they may be satisfying some need of their own. Sharing information rather than giving advice allows the individual to decide for himself or herself how to use it. Good feedback is clear and well timed. In general, immediate feedback is most useful; however, excellent feedback presented at an inappropriate time may do more harm than good. Finally, following feedback with time for the receiver to ask questions or to receive clarification is important.

Although it is important to provide feedback, receiving feedback from employees can help leaders avoid making costly mistakes. Most of the time, employees provide valid suggestions and new ideas that leaders may not have considered. Not only might new ideas take hold, but when employees actively participate in meaning making (find benefits in a new process), it increases the likelihood that they will accept the changes being made (Sonenshein & Dholakia, 2014).

> By openly requesting feedback, a leader demonstrates that he or she values employee input; it also provides the leader with insight into the potential of the health system for embracing the chosen professional practice model. Such information will provide for realistic progression plans.

Providing regular, frequent, clear, constructive, well-timed feedback to employees and soliciting responses back from them is a leadership responsibility. In fact, ongoing dialog with RN staff, unified by the mutually agreed-on nursing values and PPM, should be evident in leadership actions and relationships (Salmela, Eriksson, & Fagerstrom, 2011). Modified workplace behaviors are dependent on unit-based leaders' reinforcement of new ways of practice through strategies, such as praise, modeling the change by working alongside employees, appropriate use of rewards and incentives, presenting unit-based data, and sharing best practices, all methods that deliberately keep feedback developmental (Henderson, Schoonbeek, & Auditore, 2013).

Implementation Boosters

A *booster* is a person or thing who supports, assists, or increases power or effectiveness (Booster, 2015). In this case, a booster may be additional educational sessions, selected review activities, training videos, readings, exercises, focused reflections, or consultations that are conducted periodically throughout the long-term integration process to reinforce progress. They augment other implementation strategies, providing additional opportunities to troubleshoot problems, prevent relapse, activate new behaviors, and follow up. Boosters are a source of encouragement and have been found in several studies to facilitate long-term behavior change (Fleig, Pomp, Schwarzer, & Lippke, 2013; Kroese, Adriaanse, & De Ridder, 2012).

When designing booster strategies during implementation, it is important to consider their content, timing and frequency, strength or dose, and the number of strategies to be used. Content includes what will be done and addresses the important relationship between concepts in the PPM and the desired practice behaviors in employees. There should be a deliberate attempt to link these two variables. For example, in Orem's Self-Care Theory, self-care agency is a major concept. According to Orem (1991), it represents a human ability to engage in self-care and is dependent on age, developmental state, life experiences, sociocultural orientation, health, and available resources. In a health system using Orem's theory as a component of the PPM, a booster strategy might include a case study followed by a group dialogue on the factors that may affect the individual's self-care agency. This could be followed up with an individualized plan for the enhancement of self-care agency.

Timing refers to the place in the implementation process where the boosters will be offered and *frequency* includes the number of sessions or activities that will be required. *Duration* includes the time span of the booster; in other words, over what period of time will it be offered? *Dose* refers to the strength of the booster. To determine this, achieving a balance between what has already been implemented and the current burden on recipients is beneficial. Achieving this balance usually requires booster sessions to be shorter and to use a different tactic than the original strategy used. See Appendix B for an example implementation booster outline.

Booster activities can help manage the integrity of the implementation process by structuring reinforcing activities in association with concepts in the professional practice model. Keeping the underlying professional practice model and its desired outcomes in the forefront, along with careful consideration of delivery methods, helps to enrich the process of implementation and achieve its desired outcomes.

As with educational activities, it is vital that whoever is charged with booster sessions or activities continues with an excitement for learning, exemplifies the PPM, and provides engaging opportunities for active participation. Actual approaches, although usually different and shorter, should provide enough learning to expedite problem solving.

MODES OF IMPLEMENTATION

After identifying and selecting evidence-based implementation strategies, addressing *how* they will be applied is crucial to optimizing intended results. Implementing a revised way of practicing nursing is, in a sense, an uncovering of whether the process is working as intended (progress is being made) and whether it is effective (achieves established goals). For example, as the implementation process is being executed, it is important to know how many people were served, the quality of the strategies used, the amount of money expended, and whether the strategies were implemented as intended so that important adjustments can be made before it is too late. Likewise, at the end of the implementation, learning whether knowledge was improved, behaviors were changed, or what health outcomes were influenced is important to demonstrate the value of the program. Although implementation design informs evaluation (Chapter 6), it often is not considered a top priority by busy nurse leaders who are anxious to start the project. Unfortunately, when not considered, the credibility of results can be in question.

Many businesses, including health systems, decide on a new initiative and then, after a little education and communication, announce it will begin system-wide on a certain day. Although efficient, this approach does not afford nursing (in this case) the opportunity to demonstrate how the PPM adds value to the system. A better approach is to carefully consider different modes of implementation, much like intervention research, and choose a method that best suits the purpose and context. Several examples of implementation approaches are as follows:

- Whole-system start-up—similar to a "go live" date for a new software program, a whole-system start-up suggests that on a certain date, all nursing departments will begin implementation of the new PPM. It implies that all necessary education/training and other selected strategies have been completed. As suggested previously, this approach does not take advantage of learning whether the implementation process is working as planned and may affect the credibility of the expected outcomes.

- Graduated approach—as the name suggests, this method begins the implementation process one unit at a time until all departments have received the strategies identified during implementation. The advantage to this approach is that it allows more focused attention on a particular unit; but it is less efficient, more costly, and harder to demonstrate that all units received the implementation strategies as intended, all of which affects the credibility of the expected outcomes.
- Systematic implementation approaches—these are neatly organized and orderly applications of strategies that best demonstrate progress and provide credible results. They go hand in hand with evaluation methods and are most often elaborated on in evaluation design texts. A typical approach is the pretest–posttest method in which one group is observed for certain factors, then implementation strategies are applied and are later followed by a second observation of the same factors. This approach is rather straightforward but only collects data at two points in time and often does not account for factors that could affect the data. Another systematic method is a single-group time series during which evaluations are repeated at prescribed intervals throughout the implementation process. This approach helps track trends and "paints a picture" of the progress of the project. It also allows for staggered implementation processes to be demonstrated more easily, but is more time-consuming.

The control-group design is the most robust for demonstrating credible results and, although it is time-consuming, its product is most believable. Designating a certain unit or units "implementation units" and other *similar* units as "controls," the implementation strategies are applied only to the implementation units and then, using the same evaluation indicators, are compared simultaneously to the control units. Or this approach could be used with similar patient populations versus departments. This method "demonstrates" the outcomes of the PPM more effectively by reducing potential biases that could confound the results (provided the implementation and control unit patients and personnel are similar and/or are statistically controlled).

Using these types of approaches as smaller pilot studies allows a health system to "try out" implementation strategies, assess results, revise as needed, and implement again prior to proceeding to implement the plan in the rest of the organization. This eliminates costly and unintended consequences of certain strategies and allows for staff engagement in the process.

A final example of a systematic approach to implementation is the community-based participatory action method, in which two partners (e.g., a hospital and a university) conduct a joint project to advance a local change goal. This method blends action and evaluation together but requires a collaborative commitment to an iterative process of action followed by evaluation to sustain change. It does consume considerable resources and is less efficient, but has been used successfully in advancing evidence-based practice (Friesen-Storms, Moser, van der Loo, Beurskens, & Bours, 2015; Tapp et al., 2014).

> Taking into consideration how *applying* an implementation plan affects the system's time constraints, burden to staff and patients, implementation fidelity, and feasibility facilitates sound decision making.

Although implementation approaches vary, choosing a method that best demonstrates the intended results of the PPM is crucial to showcasing how nursing adds value.

ACCOUNTABILITY

Implementation recognizes that broad goals, specific objectives, and related strategies must reflect current conditions within the organization and its environment; thus the implementation committee's effort at cultivating and including other stakeholders at various organizational levels helps an implementation plan become a reality. Building partnerships with others (e.g., health professionals in the system, academic centers, consultants, other health systems) can also help build political capital in the organization. When all objectives have been developed and detailed actions outlined, assigning responsibility and expectations for completion is the next step. When assigning responsibilities, it is important to spread the obligations across the health system and among multiple levels to avoid the trap of "lack of ownership." A project of this magnitude requires ownership at all levels. Being careful to create due dates for completion so that those assigned will understand the timing of their obligations is essential. Arranging specific strategies in order of priority from the viewpoint of the patient/family and focusing on those activities and practices that bring them the highest value are considered most significant to the PPM. Once a first draft has been prepared, receiving feedback and accepting recommendations from key constituents is helpful. See the sample implementation template in Table 5.3.

The steps listed here are just one approach to implementation design. Implementation is a process that lends itself to joint leadership–staff effort.

Table 5.3 Sample Implementation Template Goal: Professional Nursing Staff Will Comprehend the Professional Practice Model

Objectives	Strategies	Responsibility	Evaluation	Time Frame
By December 2017, at least 90% of professional nursing staff can describe the major components of the PPM	1. Review evidence-based educational strategies for inclusion 2. Identify those that best fit institutional criteria 3. Select three educational activities for inclusion 4. Develop learning objectives, content, outcomes 5. Conduct educational activities for five units 6. Evaluate and revise as needed	Nursing Research Council; nurse researcher Clinical nurse specialists and nurse educators	1. Minutes of research council reflect review of evidence 2. Best evidence for educational strategies is documented 3. Learning objectives, content, and outcomes for the three educational activities are documented 4. At least 90% of RN staff on affected units attend educational sessions (attendance records) 5. Learning outcomes reflect knowledge improvement 6. Education strategies are revised based on evaluation results	Begin January 2017; complete December 2017

Often there is a joint committee retreat early in the process, several planning sessions with a strong focus on the action plan, and a leadership session to review and approve the plan. The retreat is held in addition to regularly scheduled committee meetings and ongoing work is conducted outside the meeting. The implementation planning sessions often work best when facilitated by a knowledgeable individual who is skilled in group processes, experienced in implementation planning, and who is committed to ensuring full discussion of issues but is also task-oriented enough to be able to move the process forward.

Key factors to successful professional practice model integration are planning, selecting, and ensuring accountability for those functions, activities, or practices, defined by the professional practice model and required by patients/families, that are critical to excellence, *not* to needs of the health system. Being able to perform these in a superior fashion compared to the competition sets health systems and their nursing staff apart.

When system strengths are aligned with the major components of the PPM, the value of professional nursing practice flourishes and benefits the patient/family, the RN, and the health system.

Authentic leadership that sets an optimistic "we can do this" tone enables practice model integration. Setting clear and meaningful performance indicators from the outset helps focus the process and including a diverse team of participants facilitates understanding of those connections between day-to-day work and compelling, longer term aspirations. Furthermore, frequent and transparent dialog about the model's potential impact on patient outcomes can reinforce the foundational mission/nursing values.

SUMMARY

Planning, selecting strategies, and ensuring accountability for PPM implementation requires a working group of diverse nursing professionals from multiple levels of a health system to fully capture their expertise and insights. In this chapter, the steps of the implementation process were reviewed and examples of a SWOT analysis, broad goal statements, and measurable objectives were provided. The distinction between goals and objectives was demonstrated and criteria for selecting among many implementation strategies were suggested. Several implementation strategies were posed: education, modification of work roles, workflow redesign, effective communication, and ongoing support and enrichment. Accountability for the plan's implementation in terms of assigning responsibility, prioritizing goals, and setting realistic time frames for completion was explained. Finally, key success factors, including an optimistic leadership tone, were presented.

REFLECTIVE APPLICATIONS

For Students
1. Why is implementation planning crucial to successfully integrating PPMs?
2. Describe the components of an implementation plan. Which ones require more of your understanding? Why? How will you gain this knowledge?
3. Who should comprise the implementation planning committee? Provide a rationale for your view.
4. Conduct a SWOT analysis of your current nursing class. List its strengths, weaknesses, opportunities, and threats. What will you do with this information?

5. Develop one broad goal statement for PPM implementation. Next list three objectives designed to meet this goal. How will you know the objectives are measurable?
6. Which implementation strategies would you select? Why?
7. Explain how *applying* an implementation plan could negatively affect the results.

For Clinical Nurses

1. Which nurses in your organization could best plan the integration of a PPM? How could you provide suggestions to this planning group? What forums presently exist to facilitate your input?
2. Analyze the strengths of nursing practice in your health system? Be specific and list them. How could these be used to select strategies for a PPM implementation plan?
3. Analyze the weakness of nursing practice in your health system? Be specific and list them. Why do they exist? How would you suggest an implementation planning committee select strategies to adjust for these weaknesses?
4. Develop one goal statement to improve nursing practice in your health system. List three measurable objectives designed to meet this goal. Who would you assign responsibility for these objectives? When do you suggest the goals be completed?
5. What communication mechanisms exist in your health system that could be leveraged by an implementation planning committee?
6. Name two disadvantages of whole-system start-ups.

For Nurse Leaders

1. Who in your organization would you involve in a PPM implementation planning committee? Why? What components would you be involved in? Why?
2. Which components of a PPM implementation plan do you find the most challenging? Why? Who or what could help you with this?
3. Review the criteria for selecting implementation strategies in Table 5.2. How often have you used similar criteria in your role as leader?
4. Using the template provided for an implementation plan, create a plan for improving nursing practice on one unit that you have responsibility for. How would you prioritize the objectives? Who would you assign to complete them? How would you know it was successful?
5. Choose a systematic approach to implementation and discuss how you would go about implementing a new initiative using this method.

6. How do you create "safe space" in your areas of responsibility? What signs would lead you to think that safe space was a reality? Why? What can be done to increase the perception of safe space in your health system?
7. What forms of feedback would you design into an implementation plan? Why?
8. What takeaways from this chapter were most meaningful to you?

For Nurse Educators

1. Describe how the content in this chapter can be best translated to undergraduate students and to graduate students.
2. How could aspects of this chapter best be learned? What learning strategies will you choose? How will you ensure that cognitive, behavioral, and affective ways of learning are incorporated?
3. Develop a teaching strategy for helping clinical educators fulfill selected strategies that comprise a PPM implementation plan.
4. What encouraging behaviors and reinforcing techniques could you use in your teaching?
5. How would you help students at all levels appreciate the value of contributing to an implementation plan of this nature? What teaching strategies would you incorporate?
6. How could you best help students learn the features of good evaluation designs?

LEARNING FROM THE FIELD: IMPORTANCE OF THE CHIEF NURSE EXECUTIVE DURING IMPLEMENTATION

An 851-bed hospital in the Southeast incorporated the Quality-Caring Model© (Duffy, 2009, 2013) into its nursing professional practice model (PPM). The vision was that by integrating the core concepts of intentional caring and relationship-centered care, hospitalized patients and their families would feel cared for, and this provided the opportunity to achieve the best outcomes. After implementation strategies were carried out, the Hospital Consumer Assessment of Healthcare Providers and Systems (HCAHPS; Centers for Medicare & Medicaid Services, 2015) scores, which measure patients' experiences of care and were included as an implementation objective, did not improve. In addition, there were anecdotal stories of instances in which nurses did not consistently demonstrate caring behaviors and service recovery measures were taken to address patient and family complaints. For example, a patient told a nursing manager that all of the nurses were wonderful during his hospitalization, except for one "sour apple."

Therefore, in order to garner stronger support from the nurses to consistently demonstrate the caring behaviors reflected in the model, Kotter and Rathgeber's (2005) change model was used. In the first and second phases of the change model, setting the stage and deciding what to do, a different education strategy was provided in order to influence the nurses to consistently perform according to the model. The chief nurse executive (CNE) chose the orthopedic unit and the medical cardiology unit to personally provide that education.

During her education, the CNE presented research related to effective caring behaviors to describe how caring interventions improved patient outcomes. She also reviewed some exemplars related to nurses' use of the theory to enrich their professional practice. Discussions were held to better understand how caring behaviors could be consistently integrated in the delivery of patient care. During these discussions with staff, it was evident to the CNE that many nurses became very engaged in how to integrate the caring behaviors—it became a defining moment for them in their understanding of theory-based professional practice. It also became a defining moment for the CNE as she realized that her presence, visibility, and direct support for nurses was necessary to uphold their practice changes.

Discussions on how to integrate a professional model into nursing practice should occur directly between the CNE and staff nurses in order to enhance the dialogue on how care is delivered. Other members of the leadership team also can engage staff nurses in those discussions; however, it seems to be most meaningful to hear the vision for nursing practice directly from the CNE. Over a few months, many of the nurses became able to integrate the caring behaviors successfully in their daily care of patients. They expressed that the culture on their unit was changing and they did feel that their professional practice was enriched. HCAHPS scores for those two units have continued to be positive and are improving.

The second component of Kotter and Rathgeber's (2005) change model involved a change strategy, which Kotter and Rathgeber call "making it happen" (p. 131). This strategy reinforced the desired change through demonstration of caring behaviors during daily huddles. Daily huddles are unit-based forums led by the team leader or manager. During week 1, the theme of the huddles was about the integration of caring behaviors with a focus on spending uninterrupted time with the patient.

The theme of week 2's huddle was about integrating caring behaviors of involving the patient in the plan of care and responding to unique care requests and needs. Week 3 focused on overcoming barriers to demonstrating caring behaviors. The fourth week focused on pulling it all together for consistency in demonstrating the caring behaviors. Breaking down the educational content into workable portions and discussing them on the unit facilitated learning. Other learning strategies were used to encourage the nurses to engage in implementing the caring behaviors such as observing each other and sharing stories in which the model was effectively delivered. Nurses demonstrating the caring behaviors were positively reinforced by reward and recognition.

In addition to revised learning strategies, work has been accomplished to redesign the recruitment process to integrate the concepts of the Quality-Caring Model, so that candidates are screened for caring behaviors before they are considered for employment. Performance expectations related to caring behaviors have been incorporated into the nurses' performance appraisal tool and are reviewed annually. In addition, redesign of the leadership institute for mangers is being accomplished so that management behaviors will better support the integration of the model.

Janet Fansler

LEARNING FROM THE FIELD: INNOVATIVE IMPLEMENTATION CALLS

In January 2014, the first creating authentic relationships everyday (CARE) calls began as an implementation strategy at Novant Health Prince William Medical Center in Northern Virginia. This weekly 30-minute call includes participation from leadership, nursing staff, and support services within the facility. Story telling is used on the call as a powerful and creative approach to engage staff and leaders to share experiences about creating remarkable patient experiences and commitment to engage in compassionate and caring relationships, supporting Duffy's Quality-Caring Model, the theoretical foundation of the PPM.

Initiated by the senior director of nursing, each call has a different theme to encourage stimulating, heartfelt conversation and is used as a strategy to enculturate positive change. Staff nurses share what is important to patients, patients' concerns and needs, and how they addressed them during their hospital stay. An example of an e-mail preparing the team for the weekly call is provided (Figure 5.2).

Bringing the "heart" to healthcare.............what does that really look like?

What do you feel with your heart?

> And all your children will stretch out their hands
> And pick up the cripled man

.......Leeland

Who have you taken hold of and lifted up that needed your attention, your compassion, your empathy?

Team—stay with me here, I know we have gone from data to tough questions last week and now we are looking into your heart!

We can do this, let's have a heartfelt discussion on Thursday with you and your staff; staff are key here please bring them to this call.

Thank you for all you do.

Polly Roush, MSN, RN | Senior Director, Nursing
Novant Health Prince William Medical Center

Figure 5.2 Example e-mail invitation to weekly CARE calls from a senior director of nursing.

These CARE calls are evidence of taking the theoretical foundation of the PPM from paper to relevancy. Leadership and staff members share and hear interesting and motivating stories of caring relationships for the patient, caregivers, and community. The stories of compassionate care move, inspire, and influence all of us!

Polly Roush

REFERENCES

Andrews, K. (1971). *The concept of corporate strategy*. Homewood, IL: R. D. Irwin.

Anseel, F., & Lievens, F. (2007). The mediating role of feedback and acceptance in the relationship between feedback and attitudinal and performance outcomes. *International Journal of Selection and Assessment, 17*, 363–376.

Belschak, F. D., & Den Hartog, D. N. (2009). Consequences of positive and negative feedback: The impact of emotions and extra-role behaviors. *Applied Psychology and International Review, 58*(2), 274–303.

Bluestone, J., Johnson, P., Fullerton, J., Carr, C., Alderman, J., & Bon Tempo, J. (2013). Effective in-service training design and delivery: Evidence from an integrative literature review. *Human Resources for Health, 11*, 51. Retrieved from http://www.human-resources-health.com/content/pdf/1478-4491-11-51.pdf

Booster. (2015). *Oxford dictionary online.* Retrieved from http://www.oxforddictionaries.com/us/definition/american_english/booster?searchDictCode=all

Bowens, F. M., Frye, P. A., & Joans, W. A. (2010). Health information technology: Integration of clinical workflow into meaningful use of electronic health records. *Perspectives in Health Information Management, 7*, 1d. Retrieved from http://www.ncbi.nlm.nih.gov/pmc/articles/PMC2966355/

Brixey, J. J., Robinson, D. J., Turley, J. P., & Zhang, J. (2010). The roles of MDs and RNs as initiators and recipients of interruptions in workflow. *International Journal of Medical Informatics, 79*(6), e109–e115.

Caldwell, D. F., Chatman, J., O'Reilly, C. A., Ormiston, M., & Lapiz, M. (2008). Implementing strategic change in a health care system: The importance of leadership and change readiness. *Health Care Manage Review, 33*(2), 124–133.

Campion, T., Johnson, S. B., Paxton, E., Mushlin, A. I., & Sedrakyan, A. (2014). Implementing unique device identification in electronic health record systems: Organizational, workflow, and technological challenges. *Medical Care, 52*(1), 26–31.

Centers for Medicare & Medicaid Services. (2015). *HCAHPS: Patients' perspectives of care survey.* Retrieved from https://www.cms.gov/Medicare/Quality-Initiatives-Patient-Assessment-instruments/HospitalQualityInits/HospitalHCAHPS.html

Communication. (2015). Retrieved from http://www.businessdictionary.com/definition/communication.html

Cummings, T. G., & Worley, C. G. (2015). *Organizational development and change* (10th ed.). Stamford, CT: Cengage Learning.

Dearmon, V., Roussel, L., Buckner, E. B., Mulekar, M., Pomrenke, B., Salas, S., . . . Brown, A. (2013). Transforming care at the bedside (TCAB): Enhancing direct care and value-added care. *Journal of Nursing Management, 21*(4), 668–678.

Doran, G. T. (1981). There's a S. M. A. R. T. way to write management's goals and objectives. *Management Review (AMA FORUM), 70*(11), 35–36.

Duffy, J. (2009). *Quality caring in nursing: Apply theory to clinical practice, education and leadership.* New York, NY: Springer Publishing Company.

Duffy, J. (2013). *Quality caring in nursing and health systems: Implications for clinicians, educators, and leaders.* New York, NY: Springer Publishing Company.

Feedback. (2015). Retrieved from http://dictionary.reference.com/browse/feedback

Fleig, L., Pomp, S., Schwarzer, R., & Lippke, S. (2013). Promoting exercise maintenance: How interventions with booster sessions improve long-term rehabilitation outcomes. *Rehabilitation Psychology, 58*(4), 323–333.

Friesen-Storms, J. H., Moser, A., van der Loo, S., Beurskens, A. J., & Bours, G. J. (2015). Systematic implementation of evidence-based practice in a clinical nursing setting: A participatory action research project. *Journal of Clinical Nursing, 24*(1–2), 57–68.

George, B. (2004). *Authentic leadership: Rediscovering the secrets to creating lasting value.* San Francisco, CA: Jossey-Bass.

Henderson, A., Schoonbeek, S., & Auditore, A. (2013). Processes to engage and motivate staff. *Nursing Management, 20*(8), 18–24.

Hendricks, J., & Baume, F. (2008). The pricing of nursing care. *Journal of Advanced Nursing, 25*(3), 454–462.

Hudson, F. M. (1999). *The handbook of coaching: A comprehensive resource guide for managers, executives, consultants, and human resource professionals.* San Francisco, CA: Jossey-Bass.

International Coach Federation. (2015). *What is professional coaching?* Retrieved from http://www.coachfederation.org/need/landing.cfm?ItemNumber=978&navIte mNumber=567

Joo, B., & Park, S. (2010). Career satisfaction, organizational commitment, and turnover intention: The effects of goal orientation, organizational learning culture and developmental feedback. *Leadership and Organization Development Journal, 31*(6), 482–500.

Kotter, J., & Rathgeber, H. (2005). *Our iceberg is melting: Changing and succeeding under any conditions.* New York, NY: St. Martin's Press.

Kroese, F. M., Adriaanse, M. A., & DeRidder, D. T. D. (2012). Boosters, anyone? Exploring the added value of booster sessions in a self-management intervention. *Health Education Research, 27*(5), 825–833.

Lamont, E. (2013). Understanding the art of feminist pedagogy: Facilitating interpersonal skills learning for nurses. *Nursing Education Today, 34*(5), 679–682.

Llerena-Quinn, R. (2013). Safe space to speak above the silences. *Culture, Medicine, and Psychiatry, 37*(2), 340–346.

Meeks, L., Heit, P., & Page, R. (2009). *Totally awesome strategies for teaching health* (5th ed.). Boston, MA: McGraw-Hill.

Nowack, K. (2014). Taking the sting out of feedback. *Talent Development, 68*(8), 50–54.

Orem, D. E. (1991). *Nursing: Concepts of practice* (4th ed.). St. Louis, MO: Mosby-Year Book.

Roberts, D., & Hughes, M. (2013). What do orthopaedic nurses do? Implications of the role delineation study for certification. *Orthopaedic Nursing, 32*(4), 198–206.

Salmela, S., Eriksson, K., & Fagerstrom, L. (2011). Leading change: A three-dimensional model of nurse leaders' main tasks and roles during a change process. *Journal of Advanced Nursing, 68*(2), 423–233.

Saruhan, W. (2014). The role of corporate communication and perception of justice during organizational change process. *Business and Economics Research Journal, 5*(4), 143–166.

Schlicter, B. R., & Rose, J. (2013). Trust dynamics in a large system implementation: Six theoretical propositions. *European Journal of Information Systems, 22*, 455–474.

Skinner, B. F. (1974). *About behaviorism.* New York, NY: Random House.

Sonenshein, S., & Dholakia, U. (2014). Explaining employee engagement with strategic change implementation: A meaning-making approach. *Organization Science,* *23*(1), 1–23. Retrieved from http://pubsonline.informs.org/doi/ref/10.1287/orsc.1110.0651

Tapp, H., Kuhn, L., Alkhazraji, T., Steuerwald, M., Ludden, T., Wilson, S., . . . Dulin, M. F. (2014). Adapting community based participatory research (CBPR) methods to the implementation of an asthma shared decision making intervention in ambulatory practices. *Journal of Asthma, 51*(4), 380–390.

Upenieks, W., Akhavan, J., & Kotlerman, J. (2008). Value-added care: A paradigm shift in patient care delivery. *Nursing Economic$, 26*(5), 294–300.

Zhou, J. (2003). When the presence of creative coworkers is related to creativity: Role of supervisor close monitoring, developmental feedback, and creative personality. *Journal of Applied Psychology, 88*(3), 413–422.

CHAPTER 6

Assessing the Success of Professional Practice Models: Evaluation

KEY WORDS

Evaluation, evaluation plan, performance indicators, measurement, feedback

OBJECTIVES

By the end of this chapter, readers will be able to:

1. Explain the definition, types, and processes used for evaluation
2. Describe the purpose of evaluation frameworks
3. Identify the components of an evaluation plan
4. State at least three performance indicators associated with implementing a professional practice model (PPM)
5. Choose valid and reliable instruments
6. Analyze data-collection strategies
7. Apply at least one method for engaging end users in the evaluation process
8. Develop a transparent method for disseminating evaluation feedback

EVALUATION

Although evaluation is actually conducted during and after implementation of a project or program, it must be a consideration before the implementation process is finalized.

Incorporating evaluation into the implementation process enhances the continuity and credibility of the project, improving the likelihood of success.

The goal of evaluation is to provide objective feedback that is useful for decision making or, in a more contemporary sense, to support development of innovations and adaptation of interventions in complex dynamic environments (Patton, 2011). In this case, the aim of evaluation is to provide objective feedback on the progress of the implementation process and the extent to which intended goals and objectives were successfully met (outcomes). Because evaluation is not only a conceptual exercise, but also a practical service, Stufflebeam and Coryn (2014) pose the following *operational* definition of evaluation: "the systematic process of delineating, obtaining, reporting, and applying safety, significance, and/or equity" (p. 14). Two forms of evaluation are typically described: formative and summative.

Formative evaluation is a learning process that is intended to provide feedback on a project's progress in order to assess what more might be done to advance such progress (Bennett, 2011), providing frequent opportunities for continuous improvement. As such, the evidence obtained from formative evaluation helps to determine whether the project was implemented as planned, whether the number of recipients included reached established targets, and to assess whether adjustments are needed and, if so, to recommend them (Weiss, 1998). When performed effectively, formative evaluation ensures that implementation strategies, activities, and materials work as planned. It also helps to understand whether the strategies used are serving the target population as designed and whether the number of people being served is more or less than expected.

Summative evaluation, on the other hand, refers to the results of a program or project, and includes specific intermediate and long-term outcomes and impact measures. Summative evaluation is most often used at the end of a project to learn how well the program succeeded in achieving its ultimate goals, whether changes in participants' knowledge, attitudes, beliefs, or behaviors occurred as planned, and whether the desired goals were achieved with efficiency (McDavid, Huse, & Hawthorn, 2013). See Table 6.1 for differences and similarities between formative and summative evaluation. Both formative and summative evaluative processes work together to provide a comprehensive assessment of a project's success in meeting its goals (observed versus specified outcomes).   .

Table 6.1 Similarities and Differences Between Formative and Summative Evaluation

Formative Evaluation	Examples	Summative Evaluation	Examples
Process oriented; assesses progress	Number of participants attending a class Satisfaction levels of participants Adherence to PPM concepts	Outcomes oriented; assesses the extent of goals attained—the value of the project	Increased knowledge HCAHPS scores Infection rates
Emphasis is on the target population—the end user	Implementers, direct care nurses, patients, educators, leaders	Emphasis is on health systems—leaders, stakeholders, funders	Nursing and health system administration, board of directors, RNs, patients, and families
Conducted *during* implementation	Ongoing during implementation	Conducted *after* all project strategies have been implemented	End of project implementation
Results guide next steps; used to *improve* a project	What strategies are working/not working? How well are they working/not working? What needs improvement?	Results used to make decisions about the future	What outcomes were attained? Are they of value to the organization? At what cost? Should the project continue? Should others adopt it?
Short-term, reoccurring process	Every 6 months	Longer term; infrequent	Conducted at project's end
Internal process	Usually conducted by internal evaluators with external consultation	Internal and external process	Conducted by internal or external evaluators; benchmarked with similar external sources; subject to external review

HCAHPS, Hospital Consumer Assessment of Healthcare Providers.

Evaluation of a project or program, or a change in the manner of working, involves ongoing collection and analysis of information to inform stakeholders about its progress and the achievement of its goals (in this case, to satisfy nursing's responsibility to the health system regarding improvements in practice).

Data from this continuous assessment is used to revise the implementation process, to better manage limited resources, justify ongoing resource use, or seek additional resources, and finally, to document end-of-program accomplishments. Internal evidence generated from evaluation data ensures that goals/objectives are being met and limited system resources are prudently expended; organizations desperately need these data to make informed decisions. To gather more detailed meanings (e.g., barriers and facilitators or differences among departments) or to better understand different perspectives and contexts of the appropriateness of the implementation process, evaluation may include both quantitative data (usually used to assess specific outcomes) and qualitative data.

> During the implementation planning step of professional practice model integration, it is important to consider evaluation and even design it into the process. That way, its requirements and burdens, such as collecting data, interpreting and reporting results, are known and well planned for.

For example, the findings of data collectors could impact reliability, accuracy, and the completeness of data; the sample size could impact the use of certain statistical tests; and the preservation of confidentiality could impact access to patient or employee records; all of which negatively affect the quality of the data. Such burdens must be considered and addressed up front to avoid later credibility issues. Evaluation is intimately tied to implementation in that without it, the success of the project cannot be effectively demonstrated (and methods to improve it are left unknown). Thus, understanding and applying rigor to the evaluation process is paramount.

A thorough definition of evaluation includes: "the systematic assessment of an object's merit, worth, probity, feasibility, safety, significance, or equity" (Stufflebeam & Coryn, 2014, p. 24). The key word here is *systematic*. *Systematic* connotes a logical, orderly, consistent course of action (Figure 6.1). Such a process requires thinking about (prior to implementation) and establishing a written evaluation scheme (or plan) that allows for adequate reflection of its multiple components and consideration of assessment activities that are well designed and function optimally.

To assess the value of professional practice model (PPM) integration, it is necessary to judge the implementation's ability to do things well or at least according to some standard (merit); to meet a need with some attached value (worth); to conduct it with integrity (probity), practicality (feasibly), and safety (does not induce harm); so as to engender some

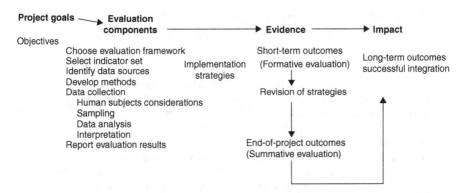

Figure 6.1 The process of systematic evaluation.

practice implications that are applied fairly (equity; Stufflebeam & Coryn, 2014). Using the more specific program evaluation standards (Yarbrough, Shulha, Hopson, & Caruthers, 2011) ensures that the ultimate purposes of evaluation—demonstrating the attainment of goals, monitoring progress and modifying project planning as appropriate, demonstrating accountability, and justifying funding—are respected. These standards address the utility of the evaluation (credibility of the process and products), feasibility (practicality), proprietary (appropriate agreements, permissions, equity, transparency, disclosure etc. are used), accuracy (quality information with justified conclusions), and accountability (documentation and benchmarking).

Another approach to ensuring a comprehensive evaluation is the reach, effectiveness, adoption, implementation, maintain (RE-AIM) method. This comprehensive approach was developed by Glasgow, McKay, Piette (2001) to be used in real-world settings. This method ensures the representativeness of participants, their demographics, and their acceptance of the implementation strategies. Calculating the proportion of implementation strategies completed and goals achieved at any point in time assesses effectiveness while also considering contextual adaptations of the strategies, the time required to implement certain strategies, and resources consumed in its analysis. Furthermore, RE-AIM allows benchmarking to similar systems to add perspective and uses qualitative data to capture facilitators, barriers, and other contextual issues.

It also considers long-term delivery of the project by examining the extent to which the PPM becomes part of routine practice and estimates efficiency by examining costs. The evaluation of a PPM integration project withdraws assets from health systems in terms of human and supply resources that must be taken into account prior to start-up.

Most decisions about maintaining a project long term are influenced, not only by the overall impact of a project, but also by its costs.

> In this situation, systematic monitoring of how *well* the implementation process is meeting important objectives (e.g., exceeds that of similar organizations or a national average); addresses the original need of the professional practice model (e.g., in terms of improving some patient factors); uses accurate information to reach defensible conclusions; is efficient; and is measured in an inclusive, ethical, practical, safe, and fair manner that provides the best evidence for formulating responsible revisions (if necessary) so that the ultimate success of the project can be realized, affords *optimum integration of the professional practice model.*

This last point—best possible integration over the long term—is most significant for health systems today as they struggle to invest in what seems like endless, continuous changes and programs.

From this perspective, designing a comprehensive and systematic evaluation plan, while simultaneously adhering to evaluation standards, should be cohesively assimilated with the implementation process. Assistance from a credible internal professional or external consultant with expertise in project evaluation who applies a monitoring and evaluation framework to the process can assist greatly with identifying evaluation components, contemplating planned activities and feedback mechanisms, and determining whether they are indeed the most appropriate ones to execute.

MONITORING AND EVALUATION FRAMEWORKS

A clear blueprint from which to monitor and evaluate the integration of a PPM facilitates a more complete understanding of the project's goals and objectives, shows the relationships among the many strategies that were developed for implementation, and describes how contextual factors may affect successful integration. Some questions to ponder prior to choosing a monitoring and evaluation framework include:

- Does the framework help to inform the progress of the project (e.g., is it useful)?
- Does the framework point to specific information that is needed to learn whether implementation strategies are being executed in the way they were planned (e.g., does it facilitate selection of indicators)?
- Does the framework clarify how to assess the results, impact, and success of the project?

- Does the framework provide a structure for determining whether the expected objectives and implementation goals were accomplished?
- Does the framework suggest competencies and responsibilities of evaluators (e.g., who is best to lead and actively participate in the evaluation)?
- Does the framework suggest sources of information?
- Does the framework account for the context of the project?
- Is the framework practical (does it use resources wisely)?
- Does the framework promote integrity, flexibility, robustness, and inclusiveness?

Determining which framework is suitable for a specific health system is difficult and some organizations prefer to combine aspects of several frameworks for a more individualized approach. Selection of the evaluation framework that best suits the implementation strategies and responds to institutional requirements is the best approach. Four popular evaluation frameworks that are used to assess the progress and outcomes of large projects/programs are described in what follows. However, they do not represent the totality of possible frameworks from which to choose.

Goals-based evaluation (GBE), a classic framework in the literature on organizational evaluation, reports evaluation results assessed only in relation to predetermined goals. The term *goals* in this approach is used broadly to include objectives, performance targets, and expected outcomes derived from an implementation plan. The goals-based approach to evaluation was developed by Tyler (1942) and has continued to evolve.

GBE focuses on the degree to which the program met its predefined goals, whether they were met on time, and, in some cases, how (or whether) goals be changed in the future. A key strength of this model is the determination of whether results align with goals. Obviously, employing the GBE framework is only useful if the goals of the project were clear in the first place, if there is consensus about them, and if they are time bound and measurable. It is also relatively simple compared to other approaches. However, it introduces bias by disregarding consequences and unintended effects as well as whether the original goals were valid. In addition, it reports findings at the end of a project, essentially eliminating the improvement benefits of formative evaluation.

To help mitigate these limitations, the goal-free evaluation (GFE) framework was designed to prevent bias by avoiding the risk of overlooking unintended results (Scriven, 1991). Instead, observations of actual processes and outcomes are made and used to assess *all* the anticipated effects of a project, providing a limitless profile. Scriven argued that, because almost all projects either fall short of their goals or overachieve them, evaluating predetermined goals may be a waste of time. GFE may be less costly to apply and is flexible, but it is prone to evaluator bias and less likely to intentionally assess the project goals because it is not explicitly centered on those goals. It also may require evaluators to do and think more. Although this framework seems simpler, many believe its limitations outweigh its advantages.

Occasionally the GBE and GFE are combined by having the GB and GF evaluators design and conduct their evaluations independently and then synthesize their results. Interpretation involves assessing the results, including whether conclusions support or contradict each other. Both sets of evaluators (possibly with key stakeholders) then weigh the data from both approaches to make an evaluative conclusion. A more theoretical evaluation framework is presented in the text that follows.

A logic model is a diagram that paints a picture of how a project is supposed to work by expressing the thinking behind a plan, that is, the rationale for the plan.

A logic model describes the overall inputs, the connections between project strategies and the anticipated short-term, intermediate, and long-term outcomes (Knowlton & Phillips, 2013). When implemented well, logic models often become reference points for participants by pointing them in the right direction, clarifying the strategy of the evaluation, reminding them of targeted goals and timelines for completion, explaining the project to others, and suggests ways to organize and prepare reports.

A logic model is created by the actual team responsible for completing the evaluation and usually is depicted in a diagram for ease of understanding (Figure 6.2). This framework shows the relationship between the context (the environment) and the inputs, processes, and outcomes of an integration project. There is no "one way" to present these processes; rather, the elements are simply ordered or mapped in a logical manner with the results clearly depicted at the end. It should be simple enough to be understood, yet contain enough degree of detail so that fundamental elements are present. Usually a goal statement is listed first, followed by more specific objectives, implementation strategies, formative and summative evaluation measures, and finally the outcomes. Context or organizational factors that can affect the attainment of outcomes can be listed anywhere. Explicit links (shown by arrows or dotted lines) between components should be clearly evident to avoid confusion. When implementation processes are well written with measurable objectives,

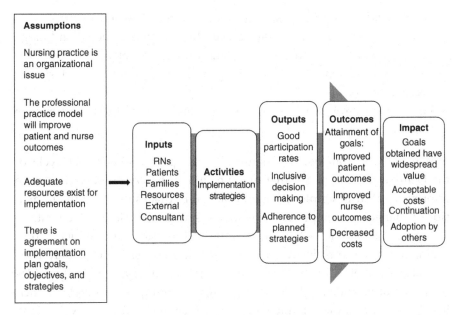

Figure 6.2 Sample logic model for a PPM integration project.

logic models essentially become a visual representation of the fundamental components of implementation with additional evaluation measures added.

> A strong rationale for using theory-based evaluation is that it offers a number of ways of carrying out an analysis of the logical or theoretical consequences of a project or program, and focuses on shared understandings of project goals and strategies, increasing the likelihood of attaining desired outcomes.

Limitations of this evaluation framework, however, include time requirements and the heavy emphasis on objective measurement, leaving less room for more qualitative data.

The Centers for Disease Control and Prevention's (CDC; 2011) well-established process for program evaluation includes six steps:

1. Engage stakeholders (those involved in project operation, including those affected by the project).
2. Describe the process (the expected goals and objectives, strategies, resources, context, and evaluation framework).
3. Focus the design (consider the purpose, users, uses, questions, methods, and agreements).

4. Gather evidence (indicators, sources, quality, quantity, and logistics).
5. Justify conclusions (link conclusions to the evidence gathered and judge them against agreed-on implementation goals and objectives; compare conclusions to existing standards, professional literature, and similar organizations).
6. Ensure use (through reporting and dissemination methods that engage stakeholders).

This evaluation framework is similar to the plan–do–check–act cycle of the Deming method (1950) that many health systems use for performance improvement. It is simple, clear, and factual but lacks focus on the human side of change, the competence of evaluators, or leadership involvement.

Stufflebeam's (1966) Context, Inputs, Process, and Product (CIPP) evaluation framework is one of the most comprehensive and widely used evaluation models. Unlike others, the CIPP framework systematically guides both evaluators and stakeholders in posing relevant questions and conducting assessments at the beginning of a project (context and input evaluation), while it is in progress (input and process evaluation), and at its end (project outcomes evaluation). This approach serves to improve and achieve accountability through a "learning-by-doing" approach (Zhang et al., 2011). It is especially relevant for guiding evaluations of programs, projects, personnel, products, institutions, and evaluation systems (Stufflebeam, 2003). The CIPP model is thorough, attends to the context, helps identify needs at the beginning of a project, monitors and documents a project's process and potential procedural barriers, provides feedback regarding the extent to which planned activities are carried out, guides staff on how to modify and improve the program plan, assesses the degree to which participants can carry out their roles, and identifies needs for project adjustments. Finally, it measures, interprets, and judges intended and unintended outcomes and interprets the positive and negative effects the program had on its target audience (Mertens & Wilson, 2012; Zhang et al., 2011). The CIPP framework applies a combination of methodological techniques to ensure all outcomes are noted and assists in verifying evaluation findings (Stufflebeam & Coryn, 2014).

The CIPP evaluation framework advocates involving stakeholders (in fact, it suggests engaging them and seeking them out); requires evaluators to study the feasibility and potential results of a project prior to implementation; and considers the institutional context, including the impact of individual personalities and the importance of the prevailing organizational climate.

One disadvantage may be the time necessary to carry out the CIPP model. Nevertheless, it is a worthy framework for systematic evaluation of PPM integration.

Although the frameworks presented here have been well applied and remain relevant, many evaluators are beginning to question whether evaluating innovation (or change) is best conducted using these traditional methods.

> The ability of a workforce to change practice in line with a professional practice model often involves constantly searching for what is working, the use of data to inform that search, and then altering approaches or changing direction as new ideas present themselves.

To do this, waiting for end-of-project outcomes reports is not seen by some as that valuable. Instead, newer views consider that continuous data collection, analysis, and interpretation be used "on the fly" to inform adjustments in implementation strategies. Furthermore, rather than the evaluators communicating results to those on the front lines, direct care professionals become active participants in the evaluation process, ensuring that their real needs and those of the patient/family are recognized and addressed. In this manner, professional evaluators, project staff, clinical staff, and project beneficiaries (e.g., patients and families and sometimes members of the community) all become colleagues in an ongoing effort to integrate the PPM into clinical practice.

THE COMPONENTS OF EVALUATION

Using an established or customized framework, an evaluation plan consists of a performance indicator set that identifies sources of data and data-collection methods, including appropriate samples, time frames, logistics (who will be responsible for what), analysis, interpretation, and dissemination (the provision of feedback). Each of these components will be briefly discussed in the text that follows.

Selecting a Logical Indicator Set

Indicators are ways of measuring (indicating) that progress on a project is being achieved. Using the overall goals and objectives in the implementation plan, indicators are identified that help monitor performance and best measure the predetermined targets. Setting indicators is a complex process of deciding what best gauges whether a project has met certain goals or effected some change. For example, good indicators can point to the extent to which the implementation goals have been met or whether a certain desirable practice change has occurred. But indicators must be comprehensive in order to provide the most value.

Indicators often measure tangible outcomes, but also changes in knowledge, attitudes, and behaviors, which are often less tangible and not always easy to count. Quantitative indicators often use frequencies (e.g., number of participants in a class), scores on some instrument (e.g., the total score on the Hospital Consumer Assessment of Healthcare Providers and Systems [HCAHPS; Price et al., 2014]), and rates (e.g., infection rates), whereas qualitative indicators are generally more descriptive and tend to use interviews, focus groups, and case studies.

Qualitative indicators are helpful in understanding complex processes or relationships. For example, a focus group may help to more fully understand *why* participants in a certain educational course did not finish. In health care, the structure, process, and outcomes format based on the widely used Donabedian health outcomes model (Donabedian, 1966) is often applied to develop a comprehensive indicator set. Whereas structural indicators are concerned with the environment (e.g., number of resources accessible to staff), process indicators examine the approach used (e.g., the number of participants who actually attended and completed an educational program), and outcomes indicators measure the results of the implementation (e.g., increased knowledge, an example of the actual objective set in the implementation plan [hence, the advantage of making it measurable at the beginning]).

Developing a comprehensive indicator set includes establishing a feasible number of structure, process, and outcomes indicators that are relevant to the project, practical enough for data collection and interpretation, and have the ability to detect change.

Ideally, a good indicator set will include both quantitative and qualitative measures that include the stakeholders (patients and nurses). It is important to note that an indicator set must be manageable, so a reasonable number of meaningful structure, process, and outcomes indicators for each objective are better than a large set of cumbersome measures.

Identify Data Sources

With a comprehensive list of specific indicators developed, one can begin to identify sources of data. Primary data sources are those that are directly accessed by the evaluator and intended to be collected for evaluation in a specific project. For example, using a questionnaire to gather patient information about their satisfaction is a primary source. Primary data is preferred because it is more reliable and objective. Secondary data are those data that are already collected and may be electronically stored. Using secondary data has advantages and disadvantages. It is easily retrievable and less labor intensive, thereby limiting expenses. However, it can be prone to inaccuracies or incompleteness. Although primary data can be collected through direct contact with participants using questionnaires, interview guides, or observations, secondary data is obtained through both internal and external sources. Internal secondary data is a practical source and may be more pertinent to the project at hand because those data come from within the organization implementing the PPM. For example, the National Database of Nursing Quality Indicators (NDNQI; Press Ganey, 2015) may be a secondary source that is quickly available, has been analyzed by similar systems and departments, and offers available benchmarks. Other internal data sources include billing databases, internal organizational data such as decision support or performance improvement departments' existing databases on patient volumes, various procedures, or demographic information. If these data are insufficient, external data sources may be helpful. Although a little more cumbersome, external data can provide timely and rich information. For example, federal government databases—such as the U.S. Census Bureau, the CDC, or the Agency for Healthcare Research and Quality (AHRQ) databases; local state health statistics; state health workforce surveys; pharmaceutical registries; and professional organization databases—offer excellent information that is often underutilized.

For each indicator developed, an appropriate data source or sources should be listed. Whatever measures are chosen (a combination of measures is best), there are several considerations to keep in mind. First, existing data may already be available that can be accessed relatively easy. It is important not to interrupt the routine clinical workflow during data collection to prevent negative feelings that might sabotage the process. Second, because this is an evaluation of a specific project, there may be a need for specialized training or consultative expertise. For example, often those new to primary data collection may introduce bias when administering questionnaires simply by their presence or verbal responses. Receiving expertise from a good consultant concerning evaluation and ensuring the appropriate training of data collectors is a must. Third, the validity and reliability of quantitative instruments must be ensured.

Validity refers to the accurateness or truthfulness of a measure such that interpretations can be supported and is usually reported in the literature (e.g., content validity, construct validity). *Reliability*, on the other hand, refers to dependability or consistency. For example, does a particular questionnaire yield the same scores when administered at different times? Depending on the nature of the evaluation, varying reliability estimates should be used. For example, if administering the same survey twice, test–retest reliability may be applied. Or, if multiple individuals are conducting the same observations, interrater reliability may be more appropriate. Examining the validity and reliability evidence for each measure used in the evaluation allows the evaluators to justify the use of that measure for the project, ultimately ensuring credibility of findings, which is necessary for effectively reporting evaluation results. If an existing questionnaire from the literature, (e.g., a pain instrument) is used, retrieving the validity and reliability estimates from the literature and documenting them for future use is beneficial. If a survey is designed by the organization to meet its unique needs (a home-grown instrument), pilot testing for validity/reliability prior to actual evaluation is essential. Those responsible for evaluation of the implementation process can make preliminary recommendations, but seeking feedback from others, including patients and direct care nurses, is helpful. Choosing the right mechanism or instrument to measure progression and/or success of PPM integration is vital. Likewise, if an instrument will be used multiple times over the course of an implementation project, ensuring that the process is consistently applied each time is crucial. Finally, in some cases, permissions and informed consents may be warranted.

Several options exist for identifying data sources and some examples are listed as follows:

- Surveys/questionnaires
- Interviews
- Focus groups
- Observation checklists and/or videos
- Tests of knowledge
- Existing data—records and databases
- Key informants
- External peer review
- Case studies
- Diaries/journals
- Logs/meeting minutes/participation lists

Once all the sources of data are identified and examined for psychometric properties, methods for data collection can be pursued.

Develop Evaluation Methods

Data Collection

Data collection includes the actual gathering of information to address whether the study objectives are on target and/or being met. There are many methods available to gather information, but selecting the methods that provide the best available evidence is the most crucial. Thinking ahead about how often the information should be collected and then analyzed, interpreted, and disseminated is also prudent.

> On a practical level, several issues should be considered when choosing data-collection methods. They are believability of findings, proficiency of the evaluators, costs, and the practicality or time constraints associated with the process. Of these, the first two are connected.

Results must be considered believable in order that those with responsibility for decision making accept them as valid and use them to refine the project. Thus, evaluators who are not prepared to collect complete data with accuracy can impact the credibility of findings. Poorly collected information that cannot be trusted, is incomplete, or is not relevant jeopardizes the project as a skeptical audience will find ways to doubt the findings. Obviously, the time required and associated costs of data collection are a concern to the organization, so practical data-collection methods that yield credible findings are the goal.

Adequate data collection is an important part of high-quality evaluation results. For a more complete discussion of this concept, please refer to *Nursing Research: Generating and Assessing Evidence for Nursing Practice; Generating and Assessing Evidence for Nursing Practice*, 9th Edition (Polit & Beck, 2012) or *Understanding Nursing Research: Building an Evidence-Based Practice* (Grove, Burns, & Gray, 2013). Based on the data sources identified, the actual data-collection method varies; however, sensitivity to participants' time and clinical condition (aka burden); completeness; consistency of method over time; accuracy; consideration of any confounding factors, including data-collector bias, training of data collectors, compiling data-collection forms or electronic procedures; and fidelity to the overall evaluation plan are crucial elements. Thus, before the evaluation is conducted (during the implementation planning stage), ensuring that data-gathering methods are known and well planned for ensures integrity of results. This is usually accomplished via a thorough data-collection plan. Finally, consideration of human subjects, a significant professional responsibility, is always an element of appropriate data collection.

Human Subjects

Evaluation and research are linked, but they serve different purposes. Evaluation focuses on a project or program and is aimed at improvement and determining value, whereas research more often focuses on populations and is often value free (Scriven, 2004).

> Although evaluation is different from research, many of the same techniques are used and some can risk harm to individuals, leaving the protection of human subject in jeopardy.

When evaluation involves collecting information from individuals in any way (e.g., observations, interviews, surveys, or personal health information), if identifiable data will be collected, or if the results are intended for a wider audience (e.g., presented outside an institution at conferences or in the literature) to inform others, evaluators might unintentionally violate individuals' rights. Thus, human subjects' protection review is a reasonable course of action that is a professional responsibility. Most health care systems have policies that govern this process. Although there is variability in institutional review board (IRB) policies (Patel, Stevens, & Puga, 2013), access to, understanding, and adhering to the institutional policy on protection of human subjects is a necessary prerequisite to evaluation. If there is any question, consult the IRB prior to data collection!

> Nurse leaders have a special responsibility to ensure adherence to local IRB policies and to monitor the interactions of evaluation teams and stakeholders to ensure civility throughout the process.

Sampling

Sampling refers to selecting a portion of subjects (the sample) in order to learn something about the entire population without having to measure the whole group.

Sampling can reduce the need to measure the entire population of interest (obtaining a 100% response rate is usually not feasible), but must be done in a systematic manner to correctly interpret findings.

There are many types of sampling methods, which are not the purview of this text. However, in evaluation, typically, convenience, purposive, stratified, and random sampling methods are used.

Convenience sampling is just as the name suggests: it involves the first group of participants who are willing to be measured. Although this method is practical, it is faulty in that it interjects bias. Purposive sampling seeks to get viewpoints from a particular group (e.g., perioperative room nurses) and may be useful when a specific population's perspectives are needed. Stratified sampling refers to first separating distinct populations into groups (strata), and then selecting a random number from each group. For example, to achieve reasonable representativeness of critical care nurses in a health system with five critical care units (CCUs), the evaluator might first divide the critical care nurse population into those working in the coronary care unit, the medical intensive care unit (ICU), the surgical ICU, the neuro ICU, and the trauma ICU. Then he or she randomly selects an equal (if possible) number of nurses from each of the units.

Random or systematic sampling generally is used when the evaluator wants to limit bias. In the random-sampling method, each individual in the population has an equal chance of being chosen, but through a systematic selection process, only a proportion of the total is measured. For example, if the evaluation was interested in a specific hospital unit's nurses, all nurses on the payroll for that unit would qualify. Then, through a random selection process, a sample of nurses would be identified for inclusion. Although a complete discussion of sampling methods is not the purview of this text, several approaches are available to select a relevant random sample for project evaluation such as a table of random numbers, or using the nth selection technique (systematic sampling). These methods are extremely useful to eliminate bias. However, when collecting data in the context of a clinical service, sampling can be a challenging and burdensome process.

Sampling for research purposes (probability sampling) assumes a stable population with a normal distribution of certain variables, but sampling for health care projects cannot make these same assumptions because of the dynamic nature of populations whereby distributions for certain variables change over time (Perla, Provost, & Murray, 2013). If the objective of a specific evaluation is to make statistically valid decisions for widespread dissemination to others (generalizability), then probability sampling using acceptable power analysis techniques is appropriate. If, however, the objective for a project evaluation is to learn whether progress or trends are occurring, or if some change or improvement has transpired, then a sample size that is just large enough based on past experience or expertise is usually sufficient.

> The best guide for sampling in project evaluation is to think critically about the objectives of the analysis *before* any data is collected. In general, project evaluations with a smaller number of participants require larger samples. But in reality, the size of the sample should be just large and representative enough so that there is sufficient confidence (believability) in the results to provide direction for moving forward internally.

Data Analysis

Once data is collected, setting up a process to organize the data, keep it secure, confirm its accuracy, and determine the results is necessary. Most often, a statistical consultant can provide useful expertise during this phase.

> Appropriate coding of data, establishing a procedure for receiving and recording the information as it comes in, checking for accurate and completed questionnaires or transcripts, ensuring the confidentiality and security of the data by password protection and locking cabinets or offices for storage, backing up all databases, tracking all data through a spreadsheet, and entering the data correctly into a database that is set up for analysis (e.g., statistical software) are tasks that, when conducted appropriately, ensure a good analysis.

Analyzing data is a daunting task to some, because it often requires knowledge of statistical methods. Evaluation data, in general, uses descriptive statistics (e.g., frequencies, percentages, and measures of central tendency such as means) to characterize the participants and note progress. However, when changes, improvements, and relationships among variables or differences are the desired end points, significance testing is warranted (certain objectives in a PPM integration project lend themselves to such an analysis). For example, if a unit's patient-experiences scores are an identified indicator for analysis, it might be useful to measure them over time to examine any change or improvement. Another example, assessing whether nurses' knowledge of a PPM significantly improves after an educational offering, might be detected using a paired *t*-test to compare differences in knowledge scores before and after class. Or, to assess whether nursing time in direct patient care is related to patient engagement scores, a Pearson's *r* may be used. Conducting these analyses is often complex, and specific conditions in terms of the samples used and the type of data collected must be met; thus, consultation with a statistician is usually required. Furthermore, evaluators should "consider what the intended audience wants and needs to learn from the data and then choose analysis methods that will best address the focal questions and fit the data's characteristics" (Stufflebeam & Coryn, 2014, p. 565).

The process of quantitative data analysis usually begins with exploring the data set (Grove, Burns, & Gran, 2013) to learn about its strengths and weaknesses, check for outliers, and verify any assumptions. Then this process is followed up with more complex directed analyses. Qualitative analysis (e.g., resulting from interviews, focus groups), on the other hand, usually results in narrative summaries, themes, or differences in results based on different samples collected. Analysis involves reading text, coding it, and determining patterns or commonalities. There are many methods for analyzing qualitative data just as there are many statistical procedures for analyzing quantitative data. Qualitative data analysis requires systematic rigor in order to be deemed trustworthy and often warrants additional verification.

> What is important to understand from this discussion of quantitative and qualitative data analyses is that there is no one right way to analyze evaluation data. Rather, it is related to the program's purposes and institution-specific needs, requiring some forethought and consultation so that it permits straightforward and credible interpretation of results.

Interpretation of Results

Interpretation of results is an informed opinion, or value judgment, about the data that provides meaning in a specific context. When examining the results, drawing out specific outcomes, trends, and patterns in the data, as well as any unusual or unanticipated findings, is essential in order to help others know how to use them to make decisions. Relating these findings back to the original goals and objectives helps to organize the information for ease of reporting and allows comparison to what was actually expected in the original plan. Using the PPM as a guide, consideration of organizational factors that may have hindered or facilitated goal attainment helps to explain progression.

To decrease bias, bringing the original implementation committee together to learn about and discuss the findings and their meanings is beneficial. This group includes those key individuals who can knowledgeably respond to the evidence by providing recommendations for improvement or to document goals attained and lessons learned. It provides support for continuing on a certain path or changing it and sets up the proper format for reporting results to the wider health system.

REPORTING EVALUATION RESULTS

Disseminating the results of evaluation data to stakeholders—in this case the RN workforce, patients, and families—is a necessary form of feedback that allows for active participation, generation of ongoing enthusiasm for the project, ensures integrity and transparency of the process, and drives progression.

The format for internally spreading evaluation data may take several different forms, including electronic or written reports, memos, formal presentations, meetings, individual discussions, newsletters, or report cards, snapshots, and scorecards.

In written evaluation reports, the importance of providing *only* relevant information in a manner that is clear, readable, and captures attention cannot be overestimated. Individuals tend to get lost in complex, long and irrelevant details; thus, only pertinent information presented in a friendly manner is necessary. Usually, a title page; an overview of major findings (executive summary); a short background or reference point; types of data collected, including the method followed (with time frames) and the analyses used; specific results arranged by goal; and summary recommendations comprise an evaluation report. Occasionally appendices are used to provide more detailed information not included in the report (e.g., questionnaires used or detailed analytics). Logical sequencing of findings, integrity of the evaluation process (including protection of human subjects), and conclusions backed up with evidence should be readily apparent.

The strategic use of tables, graphs, and pictures oftentimes simplifies large amounts of quantitative data in evaluation reports, but if not done with sensitivity to the audience, it can hinder the process.

Visual representation of data is a powerful tool for understanding information. For example, the audience of direct care nurses will not be interested in comprehensive tables with complex statistical test results. Rather, they would more likely appreciate unit-level data presented in tables and graphs with some narrative explanation related to how the professional practice integration project is achieving intended patient or nurse outcomes. Administrative audiences may appreciate more system-level data related to how the integration project is meeting its overall goals, including costs. Occasionally, quotes from qualitative data can be added to further clarify or explain the graphical representation of numerical information. Graphical data displays help the decision maker to gain an understanding of the underlying structure of the data. For example, the distribution of certain variables, relationships noted, and trends in data can be gleaned from charts and graphs. Although graphical data displays are powerful tools for communicating information, presenting the data clearly and accurately requires graphical competence. Graphical competence is the process of transmission of information at the capability and interest level of the viewer (Henry, 1995). It involves selecting meaningful data; the actual production of the data displays using density appropriate to the audience; applying suitable labels, legends, and titles to enhance clarity; and helping the audience understand the conclusions of the data presented (e.g., actual amounts, central tendencies, or patterns). Edward Tufte's (1997, 2006) work on displaying data is an excellent resource (www.edwardtufte .com/tufte). Furthermore, several software tools are now available to assist with graphical presentations, generating more appeal that engages the audience and ultimately generates diversity of ideas for improvement.

Timing of evaluation results is both a practical issue and crucial for maintaining momentum of an integration project. Thus, more formal written reports may be provided less often (e.g., quarterly or annually), whereas informal results may be spread more often—monthly or even weekly (depending on the objective), using other forms of presentation. For example, in the context of staff meetings or workshops, a less formal but serious stance might be used, with simple details presented in a clear manner. Visuals are helpful, but engaging the audience with questions or meaningful activities, and even using humor generates a more participatory learning environment. Finally, verbal presentation should be brief—busy clinicians often cannot be away from the practice environment for long periods. After a verbal presentation, asking the audience for feedback may provide some anecdotal evidence of whether the results were understood and whether any suggestions for improvement could be gleaned. This allows for participation by those providing care, an important aspect of change management (Fuchs & Puska, 2014). Presenting and reinforcing evaluation results in this manner demonstrates transparency, facilitates consensus building, and suggests ownership of evaluation findings.

Engaging Stakeholders in Evaluation

Because direct care nurses will be primarily charged with applying the PPM, they will naturally be interested in the evaluation, and will desire input into what will be done with the results. Other stakeholders include nursing administration, project staff, executive-level administrators, other leaders from the organization whom the project affects, and persons who will make decisions about the program (e.g., educators). Although they may not know it, patients and families will reap the benefits (or harms) resulting from the PPM, so gathering their input throughout the process is clearly relevant. Although no evidence exists for the best ways to engage patients and families in evaluation, most research studies show that focus groups, interviews, surveys, serving on an advisory council, or attending regular meetings with researchers are the approaches used most often (Domecq et al., 2014). Regular involvement of stakeholders in the evaluation process, although beneficial to project outcomes, often presents challenges.

Stakeholders can help (or hinder) an evaluation because they are more likely to support the evaluation recommendations if they are involved in the evaluation process. Conversely, without stakeholder support, evaluation results may be ignored, criticized, resisted, or even sabotaged (CDC, 2011). For example, regularly soliciting stakeholder insights or preferences about data collection may lead to a more complete data set. However, no input from stakeholders in the evaluation process may lead to negative attitudes about the evaluation recommendations, resulting in poor adherence to the suggested actions. Thus, giving priority to feedback from stakeholders who are responsible for implementation of the model, who will advocate for it, or who are funding continuation of it, may likely lead to more relevant and actionable results, thereby helping to ensure the project's success (AHRQ, 2011).

Transparency

Transparency is defined as "the free flow of information that is open to the scrutiny of others" (National Patient Safety Foundation, 2015, p. 1). With regard to evaluation, transparency represents full disclosure of results, methods, and even strategies that are not well performed. Health systems often unknowingly create obstacles to transparency, especially related to reporting evaluation results. These obstacles range from concerns about unfairness, liability, future funding, poor explanations of evaluation methods, to closed infrastructures for reporting and disseminating lessons learned. Yet, transparency is increasingly tied to improved health care quality (National Patient Safety Foundation, 2015) and employee engagement (Vogelgesang, Leroy, & Avolio, 2013).

> Thus, in a professional practice model integration project, transparency of process and outcomes may not only ensure that the practice changes are user-friendly, but represent an opportunity for even greater successes.

If nurses are expected to change practice, access to information about the project, forums for dialog about what is working and what is not working across the system or with others who use a similar model, and availability of evaluation data will be as critical as specific implementation strategies. Possible examples of access to evaluation information include a password-protected website devoted to the project, one-page action briefs, simple e-mail blasts with information about the PPM, regular open town hall meetings, storyboards, and other reports. Using such ideas will create an open, inviting environment for the generation of new ideas and innovative actions. Such a transparent culture, where sharing of powerful information is the norm, facilitates actionable insights and encourages active participation.

THE VALUE OF SYSTEMIC EVALUATION: BUILDING A CULTURE OF ACCOUNTABILITY

Without a thorough understanding of evaluation (in the context of an integration project) insensitive and sometimes harmful consequences can occur. It is not uncommon to see health systems using "home-grown" questionnaires with no knowledge of their reliability and validity. Likewise, oftentimes these instruments have been developed from an adult, Caucasian, middle-class perspective without input from patients or families. Moreover, the constant focus on reimbursable outcomes (e.g., HCAHPS scores, readmission rates, quality measures) takes the attention away from process, such that ongoing formative assessment of progress (e.g., variation among hospital units) often becomes murky. Many excuses exist for not following a systematic evaluation plan, including not enough time, the "we do evaluation this way" mantra, lack of methodological skills, lack of sharing of evaluation results with direct care employees (data is kept close to the chest), evaluation results are not *used* to change practice, and stakeholder participation is not sought. Yet, integration of a PPM is a culture change that requires multiple strategies and resources. Isn't generating high-quality evaluation data the most responsible way to demonstrate the progress and outcomes of the PPM? Doesn't nursing have an obligation to clearly report these data in order to demonstrate their ongoing commitment to the PPM, make informed (evidence-based) decisions, and share in any consequences (both good and bad) as a result of the strategies implemented?

Professional accountability has been defined as "taking responsibility for one's nursing judgments, actions, and omissions as they relate to life-long learning, maintaining competency, and upholding both quality patient care outcomes and standards of the profession while being answerable to those who are influenced by one's nursing practice" (Krautscheid, 2014, p. 46).

Because nursing leaders have accountability for nursing issues on a larger scale, including sensitivity to both quality and financial consequences, linking project implementation strategies to results and demonstrating the contribution of nursing to the larger health system is a major aspect of their role.

Setting clear expectations, following through, communicating progress, validating outcomes, and owning the outcomes of a PPM integration project are leader responsibilities that set the tone for a culture of accountability.

Although systematic evaluation can appear to be a formidable process, it builds capacity for accountability in a health system by helping individuals "learn from the practice" (Schon, 1983). Learning from practice is a more informal approach to professional learning in which employees analyze and improve their own practice behaviors through individual and group reflection and self-improvement.

The evaluation process itself can be used as a forum for dialogue and learning. Ideas and generalizations produced by evaluation data (internal evidence) can be used to stimulate innovation, inquiry, and legitimatize the seriousness of the professional practice model.

Oftentimes, measures used during a project evaluation become standard practice long after a project is completed. And, based on the amount of transparency demonstrated, a strategy that no one prioritized earlier may become more visible (Mickwitz, 2003). For example, through access to data, a team of employees working together can speak about the results, and from their unique vantage point visualize a new or refined strategy that might make all the difference in the plan's progress. Finally, others in the organization may appreciate the evaluation results so much that they begin to evaluate in a similar manner, often asking for help from the PPM implementation team! For the profession, systematic evaluation findings at one organization, if disseminated widely, can help others replicate the implementation plan, adding more value to patients, nursing, and the health system.

To resolve many of the unknowns associated with changing nursing practice through a PPM, leaders and end users must learn; such learning can occur through systematic evaluation. The evaluation process itself provides structure, a time frame, and methods to help determine whether the objectives set up through the implementation plan are being met. Short term, any changes recommended as a result of formative evaluation should uphold the goals articulated in the longer term implementation process. In some cases, recommended changes in strategies cannot be accommodated; thus, some changes in the original implementation process may be called for. In this case, a repeat of part or all of the implementation planning process (see Chapter 5) will help to get the system back on course and in a position to meet its goals. Using evidence in this fashion helps to address challenges earlier in the process by providing information that can change strategy and improve commitment to the articulated goals.

Using evaluation data to change implementation strategies increases understanding of the PPM, enhances organizational communication by providing a forum for understanding why the intended results were or were not successful, and raises the bar for *using* evidence in decision making.

> Considering evaluation a fundamental part of integrating the professional practice model at the outset, securing commitment and resources, and involving stakeholders in the process fosters a learning environment—learning from the practice—that will endure long after the integration is complete.

Using evaluation findings to make decisions (i.e., living it) models and embeds the habit of using evidence in everyday practice, thereby sparking a culture of accountability that enhances professional practice. It is important to remember that because integrating a PPM occurs in the context of a larger health system, it may force changes on the organization as a whole. Thus, some blending may occur over time producing synergistic, creative, and mutually rewarding learning cultures where evidence-based practice improvement becomes more of an acceptable norm.

SUMMARY

Evaluation of PPM integration projects involves a complete understanding of the evaluation process, including its purpose and multiple components. In this chapter, two types of evaluation were described: formative and summative. Evaluation data standards and evaluation frameworks were discussed with examples provided that are pertinent to health care systems. The advantages and disadvantages of four distinct evaluation frameworks were presented and questions for selecting among them were suggested. The components of evaluation, such as the indicator set, sources of data, and evaluation methods, were presented with suggestions and examples. Reporting of evaluation results, including written and verbal forms, engaging stakeholders, and transparency of results, were also presented. Finally the value of systematic project evaluation in terms of building capacity for practice-based learning, organization communication, and accountability was presented.

REFLECTIVE APPLICATIONS

For Students
1. What is the purpose of evaluation?
2. Describe the components of a project evaluation. Which ones require more of your understanding? Why? How will you gain this knowledge?
3. Discriminate between formative and summative evaluation. Provide an example of each.
4. Provide a rationale for developing the evaluation plan together with a class on project implementation. How will you use this in your career?
5. Consider a specific goal you have related to improving patient care. Develop a logic model to evaluate this goal.
6. Build a case for choosing the GFE framework to evaluate a PPM integration project. How would it enhance the results?
7. Design one structure, one process, and one outcomes indicator for the objective: by 2018, at least a 5% increase in patient engagement at discharge will be measured.
8. Where would you find data sources for these indicators?

9. Does project evaluation need IRB approval? Why or why not?
10. How would you determine the sample size for an evaluation of nurses' knowledge?
11. Design a one-page evaluation report template. How would data be displayed? What narrative would be presented? To whom would it be disseminated?
12. What methods would you advocate for engaging staff nurses in the evaluation process? Defend you answer.

For Clinical Nurses
1. Which nurses in your organization could best facilitate evaluation of a PPM integration project? How could you engage in this group? What forums presently exist to facilitate your engagement?
2. Analyze the understanding of systematic evaluation in your health system? Be specific—what are the strengths and limitations? List them. How could the strengths be leveraged to conduct project evaluation? How could the limitations be improved?
3. What evaluation framework does your organization use? How do you know? Where could you find out? How apparent are the evaluation standards in your organization?
4. What indicators does the nursing department at your organization currently report on? What are their latest results as they relate to your department? What are you doing to improve your unit's progress/improvement in this performance measure?
5. What feedback mechanisms exist at your health system that could be leveraged by a project evaluation committee?
6. Suggest three methods for improving the transparency of evaluation results for your health system.
7. Describe the policy for human subjects in your health system? How can you access it? What is the process for IRB approval?

For Nurse Leaders
1. Who in your organization would you recommend participate in the evaluation of a PPM integration project? Why? What components would you be involved in? Why?
2. Which components of a PPM project evaluation do you find the most challenging? Why? Who or what could help you with this?
3. Review the questions to consider before selecting an evaluation framework. How often have you used similar questions in your role as leader?

4. Using the discussion about indicator sets, design at least three indicators relevant to PPM integration. What are their data sources? What measures would you choose to evaluate their progress? Who would you assign to collect the data? Why? How would you determine the required sample?

5. Who in your organization can you turn to for advice on evaluation methods and statistical technique? Can you identify someone outside the organization whom you could ask for advice?

6. How do you ensure transparency of results in your areas of responsibility? What signs would lead you to think that transparency is already a reality? Why? What can be done to increase the perception of data transparency in your health system?

7. What forms of feedback do you use to report evaluation/performance improvement data? How do you engage direct care nurses? After reading this chapter, would you change this approach? Why or why not?

8. What are the main benefits and some of the consequences of using existing information for judging an integration project?

9. As a nurse leader, how do you ensure that appropriate human subject approvals are sought?

10. Argue the pros and cons of investing time and resources to design a systematic evaluation for integrating a PPM.

11. Discuss issues that evaluation reports must consider when disseminating results to direct care nurses.

For Nurse Educators

1. Describe how the content in this chapter can be best translated to undergraduate and graduate students.

2. How could aspects of this chapter best be learned? What learning strategies will you choose? How will you ensure that cognitive, behavioral, and affective ways of learning are incorporated?

3. Develop a teaching strategy for helping nurse leaders better understand evaluation methods.

4. Protection of human subjects during project evaluation is rather ambiguous. How could you help students better understand their obligations for human subject approval related to performance improvement/project evaluation?

5. How would you help students at all levels appreciate the value of engaging in project evaluation? What teaching strategies would you use?

6. What methods do you think would help students at all levels to create and interpret meaningful evaluation results?

7. How engaged are you in project evaluation? What do you need to learn/ relearn in order to help others with project evaluation?

LEARNING FROM THE FIELD: HOW UNIT-LEVEL FORMATIVE DATA IMPROVED IMPLEMENTATION PROGRESS

Joanne, a nursing consultant, was helping a nursing department in a midsize community teaching hospital implement a plan to integrate a professional practice model (PPM). An educational program was completed and a new patient care delivery system, designed by direct care nurses, nurse leaders, and nurse educators, was being implemented. As Joanne made rounds on the units and spoke with direct care nurses and leaders, she noticed large differences in how well the agreed-on patient care delivery system was being implemented. For example, on one unit, patient white boards with the requisite questions answered were visible and completed on admission (as planned) but on another unit, this practice was followed haphazardly. Nurses' participation on rounds also varied among units. At routine implementation committee meetings it became clear that the unit leaders saw their role in this project differently. Some were heavily involved, offering daily updates and facilitating group dialogues. Others were rather complacent about the process, relying on educators, clinical specialists, unit champions, and others to implement the project. The chief nurse executive (CNE) did not address these differences with the leaders.

Over time, Joanne became worried that the patient care delivery system, based on the PPM and an important implementation strategy, would not be applied consistently and that this would affect both formative and summative evaluation results. In fact, the most recent formative evaluation results showed major variances in patients' perceptions of nurse responsiveness, patients' familiarity with the health care team, patients' self-reported pain scores, and nurse engagement, all preidentified indicators of progress.

To improve fidelity of the implementation plan and progress on the integration, Joanne decided to use a data-driven approach (and a little peer pressure). She developed a simple observation checklist with behaviors listed that represented aspects of the PPM that could be either visualized or gathered through existing records on the unit. Some items were listed as core to the model with an asterisk and considered mandatory (Figure 6.3).

She then trained two graduate assistants to observe these behaviors weekly on each unit, checking under the appropriate column whether the behavior was met or not. On a weekly basis, Joanne calculated percentage

Directions: Under each week, please add a Y (yes) or N (no) to record whether adherence to the associated element was met.

Element	Week 1	Week 2	Week 3	Week 4	Week 5	Week 6	Week 7	Week 8	Week 9	Week 10	Week 11	Week 12
*Answers to three questions documented on patient white boards												
*Open visiting hours												
*Purposeful interaction documented												
*Focused reminders for "centering"												
*Regular meal breaks scheduled												
RNs regularly participate in patient rounds												
Huddles used as needed to solve immediate problems												
*RNs assigned to patients; Nursing assistants assigned to tasks												
Quiet, soothing noise levels												
Therapeutic lighting observed												
*80/20 professional/assistive staff mix												
*Patients have no more than two RNs each per 24-hour period												
*RNs work at least two shifts in a row												
*RNs keep same assignment												
TOTALYs and Ns												
Percentage: adherence												
*Mandatory core element												

Figure 6.3 Observation checklist.

adherence overall and adherence to the mandatory items separately. She then plotted the data using a line graph on one large report for the whole nursing department. These reports were then distributed to the nursing leadership team for the monthly implementation committee meetings. It soon became apparent which units were following the implementation plan and those that were not, as well as what aspects needed reinforcement. Over a period of 6 weeks, the nursing leaders came together over the data reports and worked cohesively to adhere to the implementation plan. Those leaders who had better scores shared their approach with others and some new leadership involvement strategies were designed and applied. They were empowered by the presentation of simple data that refocused their attention to the importance of fidelity to the implementation plan. The routine report soon became an expected part of the meeting generating dialogue, sharing of ideas, and the comradery required to improve progress on the implementation of the PPM.

During this 3-year project, new leaders were hired and others left the system; yet the use of these data facilitated a focused source of discussion that kept the project on track. It also prompted a modification in the way leadership meetings were conducted. As more leaders became adept at interpreting and using formative data, they began to desire more knowledge and two even returned to school. The lesson learned in this situation is to routinely incorporate data into regularly held leadership forums to generate discussion, serve as a catalyst for decision making and new ideas, and preserve teamwork.

Joanne R. Duffy

LEARNING FROM THE FIELD: COMMUNICATION OF OUTCOMES DATA USING GRAPHICAL DISPLAYS

In 2012, at an educational symposium, the process for the enculturation of the Quality-Caring Model© (QCM; Duffy, 2009) at Novant Health Prince William Medical Center (NHPWMC) began. At all nursing levels, leaders and staff nurses immediately recognized the eight caring factors of mutual problem solving, attentive reassurance, human respect, an encouraging manner, appreciation of unique meanings, healing environment, basic human and affiliation needs; the leaders and staff clearly identified the factors required to strengthen the professional practice structure for the Magnet® journey.

The hospital-wide and unit-based nursing shared governance councils focused on the need to establish nursing ownership of those patient outcomes influenced by the model, facilitating the Novant Health vision to deliver the most remarkable patient care experience in every dimension, every time.

Outcomes Measures and Data

The dynamic nature of baseline and benchmark data progression over time demonstrates how the application of the PPM fostered nursing practice to achieve and sustain patient care outcomes.

Initiative 1: Attentive Reassurance and Healing Environment

The emergency department (ED) nursing staff focused on the Centers for Medicare & Medicaid Services (CMS) measure "median" time to pain management for long-bone fracture in minutes. Using specially designed triage questions, ED nurses were prompted to reassure and clarify their intentions and respond promptly to maintain patient comfort and relieve pain. The empirical data reflected improved pain management over time beyond the national benchmark that could be tied directly to nursing quality caring (Figure 6.4).

Initiative 2: Mutual Problem Solving and Encouraging Manner

The national Surgical Care Improvement Project (SCIP) afforded the nursing staff opportunities to advocate and influence the plan of care for postoperative patients. As part of their collaborative relationships with the health care team at NHPWMC, the orthopedic nurses partnered with the orthopedic surgeons and nurse practitioners to improve and sustain urinary catheter removal. The orthopedic nurses worked with patients and families to help them understand that, based on the literature, early urinary catheter removal prevented urinary infections and supported safer patient ambulation. Through ongoing encouragement, early urinary catheter removal improved and was sustained over several quarters (Figure 6.5).

Initiative 3: Healing Environment

The CCU is a complex environment in which patients are most vulnerable and patient safety is monitored closely. Critically ill patients are at risk for hospital-acquired infections. Central-line associated bloodstream infections (CLABSI) were previously above the national benchmark prior to 2012. The CLABSI prevention bundle and checklist was rigorously instituted and resulted in a unit-based nursing practice change tied to the healing environment component of the PPM, reducing the CLABSI infection rate (Figure 6.6).

Outpatient services data—outpatient speciality services

National database—Centers for Medicare & Medicaid Services hospital compare

Benchmark used for each graph—Top 10% in United States of national hospital quality-measure data

Outpatient measure 21: Median time to pain management for long-bone fracture in minutes

Emergency services department—has outperformed the benchmark eight out of eight quarters.

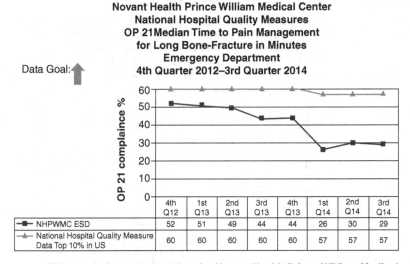

 This graph demonstrates that the Novant Health Prince William Medical Center Emergency Department has outperformed the national benchmark eight out of eight quarters.

National database used to collect this data is Centers for Medicare & Medicaid Services.

Figure 6.4 Median time to pain management for long-bone fractures in minutes. Used with permission.

Initiative 4: Mutual Problem Solving and Appreciation of Unique Meanings

In the oncology setting, patients' needs for education are key components of exemplary professional nursing practice. In particular, issues concerning patient's understanding and satisfaction regarding medications required a practice change that integrated teaching and problem solving during medication administration. The PPM—specifically, the caring factors of mutual problem solving and appreciation of unique meanings—provided oncology nurses with the foundation to better educate and answer patient questions about medications. Improvement in HCAHPS scores (Centers for Medicare & Medicaid Services, 2014) were observed and sustained almost immediately.

Outpatient services data—outpatient specially services

National database—Centers for Medicare & Medicaid Services hospital compare

Benchmark used for each graph—Top 10% in United States of national hospital quality-measure data

Surgical care improvement project (SCIP) measure 9: urinary catheter removed on postoperative day 1 or postoperative day 2 with day of surgery being day 0.

This graph demonstrates that Novant Health Prince William Medical Center has outperformed the benchmark seven out of eight quarters.

**Novant Health Prince William Medical Center
Surgical Care Improvement Project—9 Core Measures:
Urinary Catheter Removed on Postoperative Day 1 or
Postoperative Day 2 With Day of Surgery Being Day 0
4th Quarter 2012–3rd Quarter 2014**

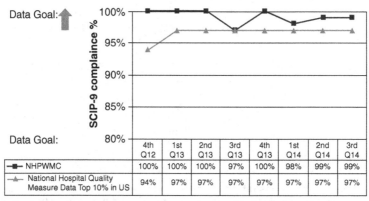

	4th Q12	1st Q13	2nd Q13	3rd Q13	4th Q13	1st Q14	2nd Q14	3rd Q14
—■— NHPWMC	100%	100%	100%	97%	100%	98%	99%	99%
—▲— National Hospital Quality Measure Data Top 10% in US	94%	97%	97%	97%	97%	97%	97%	97%

★ **This graph demonstrates that Novant Health Prince William Medical Center has outperformed the Hospital Compare/CMS benchmark seven out of eight quarters.**

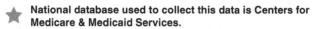 **National database used to collect this data is Centers for Medicare & Medicaid Services.**

Figure 6.5 Urinary catheter removed on postoperative day 1 or postoperative day 2. Used with permission.

Attention to these caring factors, which are integral components of the theory that undergirds the PPM, positively influenced the collaborative and nurse–patient relationships at NHPWMC, positively modifying professional practice and rapidly affecting important organizational patient outcomes. Evaluation over time, using system-reporting structures, demonstrated the translation of the PPM and supported the Magnet journey.

Eileen Caulfield

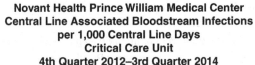

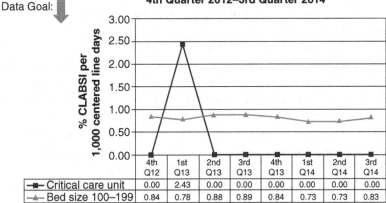

Data Goal:

	4th Q12	1st Q13	2nd Q13	3rd Q13	4th Q13	1st Q14	2nd Q14	3rd Q14
Critical care unit	0.00	2.43	0.00	0.00	0.00	0.00	0.00	0.00
Bed size 100–199	0.84	0.78	0.88	0.89	0.84	0.73	0.73	0.83

★ This graph demonstrates that Critical Care Unit outperformed the national benchmark seven out of eight quarters.

★ National database vendor used to collect this data is National Database of Nursing Quality Indicators.

Figure 6.6 Central-line-associated bloodstream infections per 1,000 central line days. Used with permission.

REFERENCES

Agency for Healthcare Research and Quality (AHRQ). (2011). *The effective health care program stakeholder guide* (AHRQ Publication No. 11-EHC069-EF). Rockville, MD: Author.

Bennett, R. E. (2011). Formative assessment. A critical review. *Assessment in Education: Principles, Policy & Practices, 18*(1), 5–25.

Centers for Disease Control and Prevention, National Center for Chronic Disease Prevention and Health Promotion, Office on Smoking and Health; Division of Nutrition, Physical Activity, and Obesity. (2011). *Developing an effective evaluation plan.* Atlanta, GA: Author.

Centers for Medicare & Medicaid Services. (2014). *HCAHPS: Patients' perspectives of care survey.* Retrieved from https://www.cms.gov/Medicare/Quality-Initiatives-Patient-Assessment-instruments/HospitalQualityInits/HospitalHCAHPS.html

Deming, E. W. (1950). *Elementary principles of the statistical control of quality.* Tokyo, Japan: Japanese Union of Scientists and Engineers.

Domecq, J. P., Prutsky, G., Elraiyah1, T., Wang, A., Nabhan, M., Shippee, N., . . . Murad M. H. (2014). Patient engagement in research: A systematic review. *BioMed Central Health Services Research, 14*(89), 1–9.

Donabedian, A. (1966). Evaluating the quality of medical care. *Milbank Memorial Fund Quarterly, 44*(3), 166–172.

Duffy, J. (2009). *Quality caring in nursing: Apply theory to clinical practice, education and leadership.* New York, NY: Springer Publishing Company.

Fuchs, S., & Prouska, R. (2014). Creating positive employee change evaluation: The role of different levels of organizational support and change participation. *Journal of Change Management, 14*(3), 361–383.

Glasgow, R. E., McKay, H. G., Piette, J. D., & Reynolds, K. D. (2001). The RE-AIM framework for evaluating interventions: What can it tell us about approaches to chronic illness management? *Patient Education and Counseling, 44*(2), 119–127.

Grove, S. K., Burns, N., & Gray, J. R. (2013). *The practice of nursing research: Appraisal, synthesis, and generation of evidence* (7th ed.). New York, NY: Saunders.

Henry, G. T. (1995). *Graphing data.* Thousand Oaks, CA: Sage.

Knowlton, L. W., & Phillips, C. C. (2013). *The logic model guidebook: Better strategies for great results* (2nd ed.). New York, NY: Sage.

Krautscheid, L. C. (2014). Defining professional nursing accountability: A literature review. *Journal of Professional Nursing, 30*(1), 43–47.

McDavid, J. C., Huse, I., & Hawthorn, L. R. L. (2013). *Program evaluation and performance measurement.* Los Angeles, CA: Sage.

Mertens, D., & Wilson, A. (2012). *Program evaluation theory and practice: A comprehensive guide.* New York, NY: Guilford Press.

Mickwitz, P. (2003). A framework for evaluating environmental policy instruments context and key concepts. *Evaluation, 9*(4), 415–436.

National Patient Safety Foundation (NPSF). (2015). *Shining a light: Safer health care through transparency* (Report of the NPSF Lucian Leape Institute Roundtable on Transparency). Boston, MA: Author. Retrieved from http://c.ymcdn.com/sites/www.npsf.org/resource/resmgr/LLI/Shining-a-Light_Transparency.pdf

Patel, D. I., Stevens, K. R., & Puga, F. (2013). Variations in institutional review board approval in the implementation of an improvement research study. *Nursing Research and Practice, 2013,* 1–6.

Patton, M. Q. (2011). *Developmental evaluation: Applying complexity concepts to enhance innovation and use.* New York, NY: Guilford Press.

Perla, R. J., Provost, L. P., & Murray, S. K. (2013). Sampling considerations for health care improvement. *Quality Management in Health Care, 22*(1), 36–47.

Polit, D. F., & Beck, C. T. (2012). *Nursing research: Generating and assessing evidence for nursing practice* (9th ed.). New York, NY: Lippincott, Williams, and Wilkins.

Press Ganey. (2015). *National Database of Nursing Quality Indicators (NDNQI).* Retrieved from http://www.nursingquality.org/

Price, A., Elliott, M. N., Zaslavsky, A. M., Hays, R. D., Lehrman, W. G., Rybowski, L., . . . Cleary, P. D. (2014). Examining the role of patient experience surveys in measuring health care quality. *Medical Care Research Review, 71*(5), 522–554.

Schon, D. (1983). *The reflective practitioner: How professionals think in action.* New York, NY: Basic Books.

Scriven, M. (1991). Prose and cons about goal-free evaluation. *American Journal of Evaluation, 12*(1), 55–62.

Scriven, M. (2004). Reflecting on the past and future of evaluation. *Evaluation Exchange.* Retrieved February 4, 2015 from http://www.hfrp.org/evaluation/the-evaluation-exchange/issue-archive/reflecting-on-the-past-and-future-of-evaluation/michael-scriven-on-the-differences-between-evaluation-and-social-science-research

Stufflebeam, D. L. (1966). *Evaluation under Title I of the elementary and Secondary Education Act of 1967.* Address delivered at the Title I Evaluation Conference sponsored by the Michigan State Department of Education, Lansing, MI.

Stufflebeam, D. L. (2003). The CIPP model for evaluation. In T. Kellaghan & D. L. Stuffelbeam (Eds.), *International handbook of educational evaluation* (pp. 31–62). Norwell, MA: Kluwer.

Stufflebeam, D. L., & Coryn, C. L. S. (2014). *Evaluation theory, models, and applications* (2nd ed.). San Francisco, CA: Jossey-Bass.

Tufte, E. R. (1997). *Visual explanations: Images and quantities, evidence and narrative.* Cheshire, CT: Graphics Press.

Tufte, E. R. (2006), *Beautiful evidence.* Cheshire, CT: Graphics Press.

Tyler, R. W. (1942). General statement on evaluation. *Journal of Educational Research, 35*(7), 492–501.

Vogelgesang, G. R., Leroy, H., & Avolio, B. J. (2013). The mediating effects of leader integrity with transparency in communication and work engagement/performance. *Leadership Quarterly, 24*(3), 405–413.

Weiss, C. (1998). Have we learned anything new about the use of evaluation? *American Journal of Evaluation, 19*(1), 21–33.

Yarbrough, D. B., Shulha, L. M., Hopson, R. K., & Caruthers, F. A. (2011). *The program evaluation standards: A guide for evaluators and evaluation users* (3rd ed.). Thousand Oaks, CA: Sage.

Zhang, G., Zeller, N., Griffith, R., Metcalf, D., Williams, J., Shea, C., & Misulis, K. (2011). Using the context, input, process, and product evaluation model (CIPP) as a comprehensive framework to guide the planning, implementation, and assessment of service-learning programs. *Journal of Higher Education and Outreach Engagement, 15*(4), 57–83.

CHAPTER 7

Refining the Professional Practice Model Within a Health System: Adaptation

KEY WORDS

Adaptation, refining, adapting a professional practice model (PPM), micro-systems, reflection

OBJECTIVES

By the end of this chapter, readers will be able to:

1. Evaluate the process of using evidence to refine and adapt a professional practice model (PPM) for local use
2. Analyze leadership's role in engaging clinical microsystems
3. Describe how the cycle of action and reflection contributes to rapid integration of PPMs

REFINING AND ADAPTING PROFESSIONAL PRACTICE MODEL IMPLEMENTATION BASED ON EVIDENCE

Using the best available evidence to inform the implementation process takes the subjectivity out of decision making, allowing the ensuing processes to evolve out of the data rather than on individual opinions.

In a project such as the integration of a professional practice model, summative data are crucial but insufficient to meet the periodic needs of end users for information that speaks to feasibility in the real world, to determine the potential influence of contextual factors, to gauge how the project participants (patients and nurses) respond, and to formulate refinements and adaptations necessary to achieve optimal integration.

Using formative evidence helps to address potential implementation weaknesses. For example, failure to implement a strategy as planned or to concurrently implement some other system-wide initiative may create unintended barriers that impede short-term goal attainment. Using formative evaluation data this way helps to identify discrepancies between the plan and how it was operationalized by identifying influences that may not have been anticipated at first. As Hulscher, Laurant, and Grol (2003) note, formative evaluation data allows the evaluation and measurement of the actual exposure to the strategy, describes the experience of those exposed, and focuses on the dynamic context within which implementation is taking place. Finally, formative evaluation data provides information to communicate to stakeholders, allowing the project to better "tell its story" *during* implementation rather than waiting until the end.

Despite the fact that modifications and adaptations are common during large-scale change projects, using data to make judgments about how the implementation process works in practice is not necessarily commonplace. Making decisions in health care, especially about professional practice, is complex and awkward to say the least. Most decisions have important consequences and involve much ambiguity, sometimes leading to disagreements, or worse, the abandonment of a course of action. In general, large-scale projects and their outcomes are enhanced by responding to various types of data that lead to informed decisions about ongoing implementation strategies, including refining or adapting them to meet the requirements of the local environment. Using data in this way facilitates integration by efficiently enabling team members to assess progress toward goals, respond to stakeholder and organizational needs, reallocate resources, and enhance original strategies. Although the original strategies provided the impetus to initiate the integration, ongoing evidence helps to improve the implementation process—by refining and adapting strategies as they are applied in varied contexts. Through this process, the implementation committee "learns" about how the strategies are received, accepted, used, and whether the stakeholders' expectations were met. In essence, the adaptation process generates new *application* data that, if used appropriately, informs the ongoing project.

> The goal of using the *refining* implementation strategies is to improve or perfect them so that any risks or barriers can be acknowledged and addressed to enhance the quality and efficiency of project outcomes. *Adapting* implementation strategies, on the other hand, refers to making informed decisions to change, alter, incorporate new ideas, or even abandon original implementation strategies.

This decision-making process is enhanced when evaluation data is applied because its objectivity allows for more straightforward selection of alternatives, stimulation of new ideas or lines of questioning, elimination of preconceived barriers such as unique patient populations, and engenders a sense of community around the professional practice model (PPM) through ongoing organizational learning.

Adapting implementation strategies is a dynamic and participatory process. It must preserve the integrity of the PPM despite differences in local circumstances that may legitimately require important variations. In adapting a particular strategy, consideration is given to local situations, such as specific patient needs, priorities, policies, and resources; to scopes of practice within the local system; and the fit within existing models of care delivery in the targeted setting. For example, in the care of children and families, family-centered care is a common overriding conceptual framework. Adapting the selected PPM to fit within this unique framework is necessary to improve uptake of the PPM.

> Being able to refine and adapt to local differences requires a willingness to critically evaluate ideas and performance as individuals and as teams.

Effective implementation committees must respond to feedback about the implementation process itself in terms of how well it is being accepted and used by nurses, how well it is progressing, how well the team is collaborating, and how the context is facilitating or hindering the plan. Implementation committees also need to consider the project outcomes in terms of their quality and from the stakeholders' perspective. Asking questions, such as the following, is necessary:

- Is value being delivered?
- Are implementation strategies feasible in the real world?
- Is integration of a reliable, adaptable PPM steadily progressing?

- Is the team working well together?
- How do organizational attributes contribute to or detract from the implementation plan?

By regularly consolidating and combining evaluation data with their understanding of the situation (i.e., insights regarding particular units and their patient populations) the implementation committee members, particularly nurse leaders, are key to this process because of the information they supply. Such information can then become actionable knowledge (as it is synthesized and judged according to its merits and yields possible alternatives) that is used to make decisions (adapt) about implementation strategies. Such decisions can take the form of remediation, tailoring implementation strategies to meet individual units' needs (such as increased education or unit-specific processes), increasing or decreasing the involvement of staff members and patients in the process, setting new objectives, and identifying areas where nurses need to strengthen their own knowledge or skills. Feedback that is acted on in each of these areas—at the end of each evaluation period and at the end of the project— helps the team effectively refine strategies and adapt to needed changes imposed by units, individuals, and patients, thereby shaping optimal integration (Figure 7.1).

Considering evaluation data in this manner requires some agility—the ability to see stakeholder value as the goal versus the implementation process itself.

Although implementation and evaluation are typically perceived as static, the context in which they function is dynamic and complex. Thus, project agility is necessary to implement strategies, to explore evaluation data, to mindfully consider this data in light of system knowledge, and to contemplate multiple alternatives to improve strategies or make actionable changes. Project agility reminds us that implementation strategies, although important, are not untouchable.

Implementation strategies are meant to be guides, allowing for some uncertainty, and should be elastic enough to permit refinement and adaptive actions such that situational or changing requirements (including correcting the process) can easily take place. Implementation committees then, continuously refine and adapt implementation processes, remaining true to the ultimate integration goals. Agile committees embrace and respond to contextual variations, are flexible and efficient, and focus on the end user.

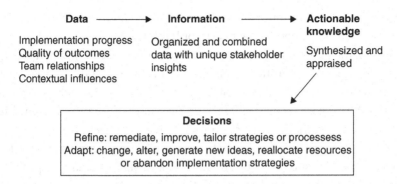

Figure 7.1 Process of *using* data to refine and adapt the implementation plan.

> Courage (to explore data, which is often an untested skill) and humility (to recognize mistakes, to improve original ideas, and alter strategies based on situations) are attributes of agile project teams.

Although such implementation committees use data to refine and adapt implementation plans, several organizational factors can impede this process. First, the accuracy and accessibility of data, together with the technical support or evaluative skill of members, can affect the implementation teams' ability to turn data into valid information and actionable knowledge. Without the availability of high-quality data and perhaps evaluation consultation assistance, data may become misinformation or lead to invalid inferences. As an example of the former, data from a questionnaire that was poorly administered (yielding low response rates) on a particular unit might misinform team members about patients' satisfaction with the PPM. An example of the latter includes incomplete understanding of the statistics used in interpreting the evaluation data, leading to the erroneous interpretation that nonsignificant changes in pre–post-test scores were meaningful indicators.

Second, the process of refinement and adaptation is not necessarily as clean or easy as Figure 7.1 depicts. Administrative pressures and internal motivation contribute to tension about evaluative data use. For example, system policies for reporting of results, as well as rewards and sanctions based on performance, create incentives and pressures to examine and use particular data, especially those related to resource use. Furthermore, the intrinsic desire to evaluate and improve individual performance may contribute to data use. For example, an implementation committee member may be inspired by the evaluation feedback and become motivated to pursue it.

Contrarily, another committee member may feel overwhelmed by the data, diminishing his or her enthusiasm for applying it.

Third, the timeliness of data, particularly delays associated with receiving results, affects committee members' ability to use the information for decision making. In contrast, the immediacy of results may enable their use throughout a project. The availability of evaluation data results at multiple points in time also enhances their utility relative to project objectives.

Fourth, the individual capacity and associated support available to committee members in terms of preparation and skill in data interpretation, formulating questions, developing solutions, access to professional development, and support from individuals who are skilled in sorting data enable data use. Obviously, lack of time to synthesize and interpret data also limits data use. Deciding how to act on implementation results requires time that most nurses do not have and few health systems allocate. Permitting protected time to regularly examine and reflect on implementation data is often missing from integration projects such as this.

Fifth, the culture and leadership within a health system also influences patterns of data use. For example, leaders with strong commitments to data-driven decision making as well as norms of openness and collaboration foster data use. On the other hand, in settings where beliefs about project feedback foster privacy, the collective examination and use of data is constrained. Many leadership implications exist as a result of these factors such as:

- The presence of data does not guarantee they will be *used* to drive refinement or adaptation of the implementation processes.
- Using various types of data collected at multiple points in time promotes informed decisions.
- Equal attention must be paid to data analysis and data decision making. These are two different behaviors, and decision making based on data is often more challenging, requiring more creativity and more time.
- High-quality data that is timely and accessible is necessary to create user enthusiasm.
- Internal motivation and system incentives may help or hinder data-driven decisions.
- Encouragement (capacity building) and technological support to aid in data use must be provided.
- A culture of inquiry must be fostered (Melnyk, Fineout-Overholt, Stillwell, & Williamson, 2009) in which nurses actively question nursing practice in a safe and encouraging atmosphere, the pursuit of best evidence is

routinely expected, nurses are knowledgeable about and committed to the use of data for decision making, diversity of ideas is appreciated, practice improvement is part of the routine, and opportunities for reflective dialogue are provided (Duffy et al., 2015).

> In an integration project of this nature where ultimate practice change is the goal, comprehensive approaches are required at different levels in the system to adapt to new ways of thinking about and practicing nursing.

Such comprehensive approaches to implementation projects are difficult to accomplish, even when there is good evidence to support them; thus, creating the environment to receive and then act on evidence is essential. Leaders play a crucial role in this process and often are active participants in the successful implementation, refinement, and adaptation at the bedside.

Foremost is leadership's comfort with and use of evaluation data to guide decision making. At times, this requires additional education and the learning of new skills, the letting go of old ways, and accepting enabling resources such as consultation, training, and instrumental assistance. For example, working directly with a statistician or evaluation consultant during examination of data can aid in accurate interpretation of the data.

> Bringing evaluation data to meetings, focusing the committee on the data rather than on opinion, asking questions, encouraging team members to create solutions based on the end users' perspectives are all important leadership functions.

This last point is crucial. Adapting PPM implementation strategies for use in the perioperative area may be quite different from those used in the neonatal intensive care unit.

> Although the core principles of the professional practice model remain, differing patient populations may require unique modifications in order to enable successful integration.

Adapting implementation strategies for use in a local context requires leaders who are able to support such local adaptations through engaging end users in cooperative decision making. In turn, they may be better able to align strategic intent with operational capacity (Ford, Boss, Alexander, Townson, & Jennings, 2004).

Encouraging and inspiring committee members to persevere in spite of the tensions associated with making informed decisions in a time-sensitive manner is also a leadership responsibility. By remaining calm themselves, encouraging experimentation, learning through both successes and mistakes, keeping the environment safe, and remembering the vision, leaders motivate committee members. Finally, the clinical microsystem approach offers a leadership strategy for evidence-based decision making that takes advantage of the local context.

ENGAGING CLINICAL MICROSYSTEMS IN REFINING AND ADAPTING TO THE PROFESSIONAL PRACTICE MODEL

Much theoretical work supports the notion that context affects organizational change, improvement, dissemination, innovation, implementation, and knowledge translation (Damschroder et al., 2009). Smaller groups, particularly those that work together over time and share similar customers (patients), have unique perspectives that when exploited, may expedite actionable change. Known as clinical microsystems, such groups are the "the small, functional, front-line units that provide most health care to most people" (Nelson et al., 2002, p. 474). As small clinical building blocks of the entire health system, microsystems are the place where patients and caregivers converge (and the work happens); effectiveness at this level translates into larger system success. When patients and RNs in these local environments are invited to use data to learn about, refine, and adapt to implementation plan strategies, the PPM is tied directly to patient care needs and daily clinical workflow, aligning the overall goals of the project with clinical practice.

> Organizing key clinical microsystems for facilitating refinement and adaptation of the implementation process may be a useful strategy for gaining whole-system advantage. Such small groups, individually at first and then collectively over time, apply evaluation data to their unique patient populations, allowing for informed improvements and/or alterations to the process that, when aggregated, optimize system integration.

Individual refinement skills are developed as new knowledge, abilities, and confidence is built, but the capacity to adapt is enhanced by leadership as leaders provide the vision for revised professional practice and continuous communication and open negotiation around the opportunities for decision making. At Dartmouth's clinical microsystem academy (https://clinicalmicrosystem.org) many resources exist to help organizations and leaders develop action-oriented microsystems. For the purposes of this text, the following strategies will provide examples of how leaders might facilitate clinical microsystems to refine and adapt the PPM implementation strategies:

- Provide regular "structured" unit-based meetings that focus on using evidence for making decisions about the implementation plan.
- Provide evaluation data in usable formats and "walk" participants through it to enhance understanding.
- Provide training on information-rich decision making (based on evidence).
- Allow clinical microsystems to seek and gain more information about their new PPM.
- Provide members of clinical microsystems some control and freedom to make decisions about how implementation strategies can be adapted for their patient population.
- Discourage negativity but accept discussions of implementation problems that are presented with possible solutions.
- Encourage communication and brainstorming to share ownership and responsibility while encouraging transparency about implementation progress.
- Remind participants that although there is loss of the familiar, practice change also represents opportunities.
- Reassure employees of their personal and collective value.
- Encourage future thinking together as leaders, nurses, and patients reinvent professional practice.
- Involve employees in the management of any refined departmental strategies and/or preparation for more organizational-level strategies.
- Assist individual employees in managing their own experience of change by cocreating appropriate short-term plans.
- Increase expectations of yourself to deal with professional practice changes, keeping quality of care and end users as priorities.
- Be upfront and honest with bad news and provide employees with positive feedback.

The clinical microsystem approach to refining and adapting a PPM in its local environment facilitates the translation of concepts into regular patterns and daily work habits of professional nurses.

BALANCING ACTION AND REFLECTION FOR RAPID INTEGRATION

Integrating a professional practice model that is lasting and pervasive in an era of cost containment requires rapid change while simultaneously adhering to reliable evaluation processes—grounded in evidence—to demonstrate the effectiveness of the approach, assess its costs, and maximize impact.

Rapid integration is dependent on balancing action (strategies from the implementation process) and reflection (based on evaluation data) in regular cycles to learn, refine, and adapt (Figure 7.2).

The implementation committee begins this process by determining the need, conducting a literature review on PPMs, and agreeing on the model. During this process, participants talk about the model, agree to undertake certain actions that will contribute to its integration and agree to an approach (i.e., the implementation and evaluation). Next, the group applies their agreed-on actions using systematic approaches in their everyday work. Strategies from the implementation process are executed

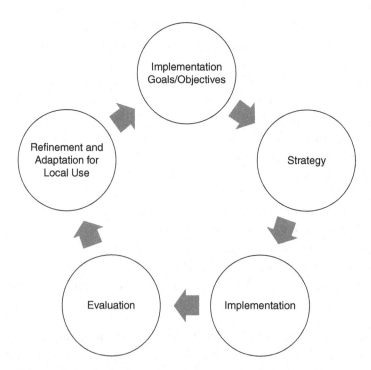

Figure 7.2 Cyclical adaptation processes of action and reflection.

and then observed, and the outcomes of their delivery are recorded based on the evaluation scheme. At first, observing and gathering data are completed in order to develop a better understanding of the experience. Over time, the participants become fully immersed in the integration process and may begin to experience it differently. For example, some participants may develop deeper insights into the PPM resulting in creative new ideas and actions, or conversely, others may allow themselves to get overwhelmed and led away from the implementation plan such that they lose awareness of the PPM and the important implementation committee they are part of.

> As the integration process ensues, participants begin to consider their original strategies in the light of their experiences and the evaluation evidence gathered. As a result, they may refine their approaches in some way, reject them and pose new strategies, or even amend ways of gathering data. A continuous cycle of action and reflection ensues in which the committee members implement strategies, gather data, and use the data to make implementation decisions.

This process of action (practical learning) and reflection (learning based on evidence) occurs several times during a PPM integration project, helping to examine experiences from different points of view, develop new ideas, and try novel ways of behaving. Through a careful examination of one's own experience and actions, gathering and analyzing key data, and in collaboration with others who share similar concerns and interests, this cycle of action and reflection helps to ensure the PPM fits with institutional attributes. However, the cycle needs to be balanced and resourceful in order to efficiently realize successful integration.

Too much time in the reflection aspect results in simple conjecturing, whereas too much time in action may represent a lot of busy work without much thought about its meaning. It may be important, particularly in the early stages, to spend considerable time reflecting in order to gather experience; and it may be important later to concentrate on trying out different actions to see how they work. Each implementation committee needs to find its own balance between action and reflection, depending on the context of the organization in which it works. An implementation committee with the ability to examine its implementation experiences with affectionate curiosity and the intention of understanding them better enhances project outcomes.

This process of action and then reflection is a discipline that helps people develop the ability to think critically. The responsibility to challenge the group, especially as it relates to the factual evaluation data (e.g., some claims may not be backed up by evidence), falls on all committee members.

Thinking critically about the implementation process is enhanced when members of the implementation committee use their collective expertise in service to the project. In order to ensure collaborative contributions within the committee, it may be useful to rotate formal leadership, to have "listening rounds" in which everyone can have a say about the topic being discussed while the rest listen, and to have regular reviews during which all committee members can say how they feel about the way the group is working. (It is also important to note that there may be people outside the implementation committee who are affected by what it does; although they cannot be full committee members, their views too should be appreciated in the spirit of cooperation and dialogue.)

Oftentimes, implementing a PPM can be an upsetting experience. The implementation committee must be willing to accept and address emotional distress openly when it arrives, allowing the distressed persons to express their feelings. Integration success is dependent on a collaborative, well-functioning implementation committee that carefully uses data to make informed decisions about moving forward.

Clearly, the processes of PPM implementation, evaluation, and refinement/adaptation can be seen as a systematic process of moving through cycles of action and reflection, taking account of experiences in one cycle and applying it to the next. But it is also about rapid movement from one way of practicing nursing to a new way, requiring a balance between action and reflection that allows for refinement and adaptation. Often this feels confusing, ambiguous, uncertain, and perhaps even chaotic, with some members feeling lost to a greater or lesser degree. Being prepared, tolerating the feelings, and supporting each other help to sustain the process.

Balancing the cycles of action and reflection is a form of practical learning, what is called by some as a professional learning community (DuFour, 2004; DuFour, DuFour, Eaker, & Many, 2006). Learning about the work takes place through the cycles in the context of a collaborative peer group that provides mutual support and challenge.

> Over time, the implementation committee may develop the capacity to shift its focus from seeking a desired outcome at all costs to the process of learning itself.

Such learning is consistent with experiential learning (Kolb, 1984) and Senge's (1990) concept of learning organizations. In learning organizations, "people continually expand their capacity to create the results they truly desire, where new and expansive patterns of thinking are nurtured, where collective aspiration is set free, and where people are continually learning to see the whole together" (p. 3).

> An effective implementation committee establishes this iterative process of action and reflection as the basis of its work through the strategy ideas it develops, the application processes it pursues, the gathering of evaluative data that it then uses for reflection, refining, and adapting behaviors, and sometimes inventing new ideas. This form of "learning" is regular, recurring, and repeated over the long term.

To be effective, leadership must provide enough structure to deal with the instability that comes from everyday human tensions concerning change, relationships with new individuals, and the lack of shared understandings related to a new practice, but not have so much structure that it paralyzes the group into inaction. This cyclical nonlinear balance of action and reflection contributes to deeper meanings about nursing and nursing practice and the emergence of a dynamic field of opportunities.

SUMMARY

In this chapter, the use of formative data to inform the refinement and adaptation of implementation plan strategies was examined. The ongoing evidence, generated by *applying* aspects of the implementation plan and then assessing results, provides rich feedback that enables effective integration. Considering the data and combining it with practical organizational insights leads to actionable knowledge that can generate decisions such as staying the course or improving a particular strategy. This continuous process of action and reflection occurs frequently over an integration project and requires team agility and leadership support. Implications for leaders are presented, including organizing clinical microsystems for data-driven decision making using local contexts as building blocks for the entire system. Finally, the developmental behaviors of action followed by reflection encourage dialogue and cooperation, which enable the development of professional learning communities.

REFLECTIVE APPLICATIONS

For Students

1. Discuss how using data enables objectivity in decision making.
2. Why is formative data so useful to project effectiveness? What formative data do you receive?
3. Discriminate between application data and outcomes data. Provide an example of each.
4. Describe a situation in which you refined your practice. What did you do? On what data did you generate improvements? How did these data help your improvement plan?
5. Describe a situation in which you adapted your practice. What did you do? How did data inform your decision about the change?
6. Explain how project agility facilitates implementation plans? How will you use this in your career?
7. List three factors that can impede the use of data to make decisions. Now create at least two solutions for each factor listed.

For Clinical Nurses

1. Which nurses in your organization could best make decisions based on data? Do they? How could you expedite this? What forums presently exist to facilitate data-driven decision making?
2. Analyze the understanding of data interpretation in your health system. Be specific—what are its strengths and limitations? List them. How could the strengths be leveraged to refine and adapt an implementation plan? How could the limitations be improved?
3. How agile are nurses in your organization? How do you know? Where could you find out?
4. How often are you asked to consider professional practice in light of data? Be specific. How often are you asked to create refinements in practice? How often are you asked to change or alter practice based on interpretation of data? What are the latest examples of practice change as it relates to your department?
5. How does your health system reduce impediments to data-driven decision making? Be specific and provide examples.

6. Suggest three methods for improving the culture of inquiry in your health system.
7. What role does leadership play in fostering a culture of inquiry in your health system?
8. Explain your clinical microsystem. What are its characteristics? How often is data presented to this microsystem? How often does the microsystem *use* data to refine or adapt clinical practice?
9. What methods would you advocate for engaging staff nurses in data-driven decision making? Defend you answer.

For Nurse Leaders
1. Who in your organization would you recommend to participate in creating refinements or adaptations of a project implementation plan based on formative data? Why? What components would you be involved in? Why?
2. Which components of data-driven decision making do you find the most challenging? Why? Who or what could help you with this?
3. Review the questions: Is value being delivered? Is integration of a reliable, adaptable innovation steadily progressing? Is the team working well together? How do organizational attributes contribute to or detract from the innovation? How often have you used similar questions in your role as leader? Name the projects. Have they worked?
4. What role does leadership play in data-driven decision making? Do you have the skills to do this? If not, where and how can you obtain them? When will you start?
5. Who in your organization can you turn to for advice on data interpretation and synthesizing evidence? Can you identify someone outside the organization whom you could ask for advice?
6. How do you ensure agility in your areas of responsibility? What signs would lead you to think that agility is already a reality? Why? What can be done to increase the perception of agility in your health system?
7. How do implementation plans currently get refined or adapted or do they? How do you engage direct care nurses? After reading this chapter, would you change your approach? Why or why not?
8. What are the main impediments in your organization for using data to judge an integration project?
9. What unique local contexts exist in your organization that may require adaptations in PPM implementation plans?
10. As a nurse leader, how do you ensure that a culture of inquiry is active in your organization?

11. Argue the pros and cons of investing time and resources to use microsystems as contextual building blocks for data-driven decision making.
12. Discuss how the continuous cycle of action and reflection ensures communities of learning.

For Nurse Educators

1. How can practice refinement or adaptation be best translated to undergraduate and graduate students?
2. What learning strategies will you use to help students understand agility? How will you ensure that cognitive, behavioral, and affective ways of learning are incorporated?
3. Develop a teaching strategy for helping nurse leaders better *use* data for creative decision making.
4. Clinical microsystems are rather ambiguous in education. What are some natural groups in your organization that would lend themselves to clinical microsystems? How could you help faculty members better utilize the clinical microsystem approach for improving student learning or to improve their teaching practices?
5. How would you help students at all levels appreciate the value of *using* data to inform decisions? What teaching strategies would you use?
6. What methods do you think would help students at all levels to balance action and reflection?
7. How engaged are you in *using* data to refine or adapt aspects of curriculum? What do you need to learn/relearn in order to help others with data interpretation?

LEARNING FROM THE FIELD: HOW A PROFESSIONAL PRACTICE MODEL TOGETHER WITH A SPIRIT OF INQUIRY LED TO A PRACTICE ADAPTATION

Janet, a bedside nurse, wanted to improve postoperative pain management at Texas Health Denton Presbyterian Hospital, but she wondered how she could change long-established and multidisciplinary systems of care. Janet's hospital is one of 14 hospitals within Texas Health Resources (THR). System-wide, the THR nursing leadership team was visionary in creating a structure conducive to a spirit of inquiry; it included new positions of doctorally prepared nurses and nurse scientists to increase evidence-based practice and provide support for clinical research. Nurse scientist positions are uncommon in nonacademic settings, yet they bolster nurses' professional practice. This vignette describes how one nurse's passion for excellence, combined with resources, such as a nurse scientist and the hospital system's professional practice model (PPM), coalesced into an actionable practice change.

The Professional Practice Model

The PPM was foundational to Janet's pain management project, which is still in progress. The THR system logo, "healing hands, caring hearts," is reflected in the components of the PPM (described later in this chapter; Figure 7.3). At the core of the model is patient- and family-centered care, surrounded by a heart made of the THR core values of respect, integrity, compassion, and excellence. Four hands frame the model and convey the components of professional development, shared decision making, the

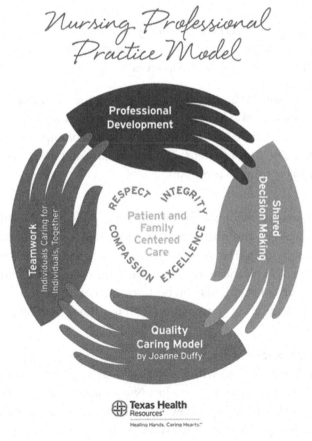

Figure 7.3 Texas Health Resources PPM. Copyright © 2015 Texas Health Resources. Used by permission. All rights reserved.

theoretical model, and teamwork. Starting at the center of the model, core values provided the sparks needed to ignite Janet's idea.

The first spark is the component of patient- and family-centered care, indicating that nurses are committed to meeting patients' needs. Other sparks are respect and compassion, critical to providing comfort and alleviating pain. Last, adhering to pain management standards of care and using research evidence in daily practice reflect excellence and integrity. In addition, these central components inside the hands in the model also framed the specifics of this ongoing project.

The pain management initiative is both an implementation of best practices and a longer term research project examining the influence of multiple factors, such as medications, doses, and surgery, on patients' first and second day average pain ratings. Project interventions included:

- Professional education on multimodal pain management for nurses and physicians
- Standardized order sets based on best practices
- Standardized patient education and a handout on postoperative pain, used on all units, starting in preop areas

Team members painstakingly gathered data from the electronic heath record over a 1-year period to track the impact of practice changes. Once data were analyzed, they could quantify the impact of improvements and use results to guide the next steps. The four major components of the PPM guided the project from its inception.

Teamwork

Because pain management is a multidisciplinary endeavor, a team of pharmacists, leaders, and nurses was created, while seeking input from medical care providers. The team met with surgeons to describe the project and goals. Based on physician feedback, the pharmacy devised an order set reflecting current standards and best practices of using nonopioid adjunctive medications in combination with traditional narcotics for post-operative pain.

Professional Development

Bedside nurses who helped with the project were eligible to earn credit toward their clinical ladder progression. Nurses and members of other disciplines contributed because they cared fervently about providing optimal care. This project prompted some nurses to seek board certification in pain management nursing. Perhaps not coincidental, some nurses involved in the project were motivated by personal and organizational factors to return to school for higher degrees.

The Quality-Caring Model©

This model focuses on caring relationships between and within nurses and their patients, families, and colleagues. Caring is the foundation for the overall goal of improving care and influences teamwork, shared decision making, and professional development. In this case, the Quality-Caring Model (Duffy, 2009) influenced how education was delivered, the process for developing the standard order set, and the patient education strategy. THR adopted the Quality-Caring Model as an essential part of its PPM during the time frame when the pain management project was being developed.

Shared Decision Making

Janet was empowered by an environment of care that enabled her to implement her ideas. She was able to initiate and sustain a practice change at the microsystem level, link it to the PPM, and use data to inform its progress. She was supported by leadership as well as colleagues across disciplines. During the year-long project, the organizational climate was in transition, with patchy progress and intermittent setbacks. However, the leadership team persisted with a council structure that empowered bedside nurses, including a shared governance council. Bedside nurses were moving from a mentality of passive acceptance and "the way we've always done it" to one of active engagement with a spirit of inquiry.

In summary, at THR, the PPM simultaneously embodies, reflects, and prompts organizational action and reflection. It represents goals as well as reality in a constant quest for excellence. In our hospital, the resources, structure, and values of the practice model served as both a catalyst and a facilitator for this project to improve patient outcomes.

Martha Sleutel
Janet Larrimore
Malika Qureshi

REFERENCES

Damschroder, L. J., Aron, D. C., Keith, R. E., Kirsh, S. R., Alexander, J. A., & Lowery, J. C. (2009). Fostering implementation of health services research findings into practice: A consolidated framework for advancing implementation science. *Implementation Science, 4*, 50.

Duffy, J. (2009). *Quality caring in nursing: Apply theory to clinical practice, education and leadership.* New York, NY: Springer Publishing Company.

Duffy, J. R., Culp, S., Yarberry, C., Stroupe, L., Sand-Jecklin, K., & Sparks Coburn, A. (2015). Nurses' research capacity and use of evidence in acute care: Baseline findings from a partnership study. *Journal of Nursing Administration, 45,* 158–164.

DuFour, R. (2004). What is a professional learning community? *Educational Leadership, 61*(8), 6–11.

DuFour, R., DuFour, R., Eaker, R., & Many, T. (2006). *Learning by doing: A handbook for professional learning communities that work.* Bloomington, IN: Solution Tree.

Ford, R., Boss, R. W., Alexander, I., Townson, D. C., & Jennings, T. A. (2004). Adapting to change in healthcare: Aligning strategic intent and operational capacity. *Hospital Topics: Research and Perspectives on Healthcare, 82*(4), 20–29.

Hulscher, M., Laurant, M., & Grol, R. (2003). Process evaluation on quality improvement interventions. *Quality and Safety in Health Care, 12*(1), 40–46.

Kolb, D. (1984). *Experiential learning: Experience as the source of learning and development.* London: Prentice-Hall.

Melnyk, B. M., Fineout-Overholt, E., Stillwell, S. B., & Williamson, K. M. (2009). Igniting a spirit of inquiry: An essential foundation for evidence-based practice. *American Journal of Nursing, 109*(11), 49–52.

Nelson, E. C., Batalden, P. B., Huber, T. P., Mohr, J. J., Godfrey, M. M., Headrick, L. A., & Wasson, J. H. (2002). Microsystems in health care: Part 1. Learning from high-performing front-line clinical units. *Joint Commission Journal of Quality Improvement, 28*(9), 472–493.

Senge, P. (1990). *The fifth discipline: The art and practice of the learning organization.* New York, NY: Doubleday.

CHAPTER 8

Translating a Professional Practice Model Into Everyday Practice: Adoption

KEY WORDS

Adoption, meaningful work, milestones, uptake

OBJECTIVES

By the end of this chapter, readers will be able to:

1. Describe the process of individual adoption of new behaviors
2. Analyze tipping points and milestones to adoption
3. Describe the relationship between the uptake of professional practice models (PPMs) and meaningful work

INDIVIDUAL ADOPTION OF PROFESSIONAL PRACTICE MODELS

Adoption of new behaviors is a complex process that takes into account individuals' intention, decision to accept, and ultimately, alters their actions related to trying out or performing new ways of being or doing in a certain setting. Thus, the environment plays a key role in the process. Greenhalgh, Robert, MacFarlane, Bate, and Kyriakidou (2004) characterized the adoption process as a series of steps: preadoption (e.g., awareness of innovation), peri-adoption (e.g., continuous access to innovation information), and established adoption (e.g., adopters' commitment to the adoption decision). Individual adoption, in the context of embracing new ways of practicing nursing, is analogous to the adoption-of-innovation (change) process that has been described by several theorists.

In this light, innovation is considered an "idea, practice or project that is perceived as new" (Rogers, 2003, p. 12) and that spreads (or diffuses) at different rates among individuals throughout an organization. Common to this notion is that adoption is a process that requires the acquisition of new knowledge, skills, and attitudes; the testing out of new ideas or behaviors in a specific context; comparing them to present practice; developing an attitude or intention toward the new behaviors; and finally, deciding whether or not to implement them (Clarke, 1996; Rogers, 1995; Wisdom, Chor, Hoagwood, & Horwitz, 2014). The various theoretical frameworks on individual adoption have different disciplinary origins (e.g., psychology, business, communication, sociology, etc.), are complementary, and add to the understanding of the adoption process; yet empirical research has not shown benefits of one over the other. Briefly, highlighted in the following text are several such frameworks from which to consider individual adoption of a professional practice model (PPM).

Prochaska and DiClemente's (1983) transtheoretical model (aka stages of change model) evolved through studies of smokers who quit on their own. The model focuses on the decision making (or intentional change) of individuals and assumes that they change behavior, especially habitual behavior, continuously through a cyclical process. The transtheoretical model suggests that individuals move through six stages of change: precontemplation, contemplation, preparation, action, maintenance, and termination. For each stage of change, different intervention strategies are most effective at moving the person to the next stage and subsequently through the model to maintenance, the ideal stage of behavior. To progress through the stages of change, individuals apply cognitive, affective, and evaluative approaches that help them make and maintain the change.

Prochaska, DiClemente, and Norcross (1992) identified five characteristics of an innovation that influence adoption: its relative advantage, compatibility, complexity, "trialability," and observability. Although this model has been used to explain health-related behavior change and encourages assessment of individuals' stage of change, it does not address the social context in which change occurs or the time requirements needed for each stage.

The social cognitive theory (SCT), initiated as the social learning theory (SLT) in the 1960s (Bandura, 1969), speculates that learning occurs in a social context that is dynamic and that reciprocal interaction between the person and his or her environment influences behavior. The emphasis on social influence, including social reinforcement, reflects how individuals acquire and perform certain behaviors. The theory takes into account a person's past experiences as an influencing factor that helps to explain how people regulate their behavior. This framework speaks to essential knowledge and skills required; modeling observed behavior; likely reinforcements that affect the continuance of the behavior; and expectations, or the anticipated consequences of a person's behavior. Finally, self-efficacy, the level of a person's confidence in his or her ability to successfully perform a behavior, is unique to the theory. Although this framework has been used by many in nursing, especially related to health-related behavior change (health promotion), it is loosely organized and based solely on the dynamic interplay among person, behavior, and environment. The theory also focuses heavily on processes of learning, disregarding other factors (such as biological or emotional) that may influence behaviors.

Rogers's Diffusion of Innovation Theory (1962) is well known to leaders of organizational change, and can be easily applied in the context of integrating a PPM in a health system. In this framework, there are five stages of adoption: awareness, persuasion (attitude), decision making (accept/reject), implementation (trial), and confirmation (adoption). Understanding the target population and the factors influencing their rate of adoption facilitates new behaviors. For example, according to Rogers (2003), innovators easily embrace new ideas and are followed by early adopters and then the early majority, late majority, and finally, the laggards, who are the last to adopt. According to Rogers (2003), earlier adopters tend to have different characteristics compared with later adopters. These characteristics offer a means of identifying individuals who could then be targeted to influence and engage others who are less eager to change.

For example, an innovation champion is often an early adopter who displays a certain charisma that facilitates adoption of the innovation, even overcoming resistance to it by others (Rogers, 2003).

Leadership's understanding of the characteristics of their employees generates a profile of potential champions that helps to identify those who can easily facilitate the adoption of new behaviors, in this case, the behaviors associated with operationalizing a professional practice model.

In a study of nurses using genetics in practice, early adopters had an overall interest in genetics, were familiar with certain genetic issues and resources, and felt a greater expectation from others to be "genetically literate" (Andrews, Tonkin, Lancastle, & Kirk, 2014). The authors concluded that knowing the characteristics of early adopters may facilitate adoption. Rogers's theory has been used successfully in many fields, including communication, information technology, agriculture, public health, criminal justice, social work, and marketing. However, it was not created for the health care environment and it lacks attention to individuals' resources or the social support necessary to adopt new behaviors. More research using the theory in the health care environment is warranted.

The theory of planned behavior (TPB; Ajzen, 1985) originated as the theory of reasoned action to predict an individual's intention to engage in a behavior at a specific time and place (Ajzen, 1991). The theory explains behaviors over which individuals have the ability to exert self-control. The key concept of the model is behavioral intent, which is influenced by the likelihood that the behavior will have the expected outcome and the subjective evaluation of the risks and benefits of that outcome. The TPB states that behavioral achievement depends on both motivation (intention) and ability (behavioral control). The TPB is composed of six constructs that collectively represent a person's actual control over the behavior. They are attitudes, behavioral intention, subjective norms, social norms, perceived power, and perceived behavioral control. The TPB has been used successfully to predict and explain a wide range of health behaviors and intentions, including smoking, drinking, health services utilization, breastfeeding, and substance use, among others. However, it assumes individual opportunities and resources, and it does not account for the environment, emotions, or past experiences that might influence behavioral intention.

Social network theory or social network analysis (SNA), derived from sociology, assumes that individuals, groups, or companies (nodes) are connected (linked) through relationships (Wasserman & Faust, 1994). All together, these various nodes (individuals) and links (connections) can be represented by a map or a network. Social networks emphasize the importance of peer-to-peer relationships in one system or explain how several companies interact with each other in a region. They help expose the channels of communication and information flow, collaborations, and disconnects among people and departments. The shape and size of social networks often influence their utility, providing explanations for behavior. For example, in systems with tighter networks, strong ties exist that encourage sharing of information and values, but limit creativity. In larger networks, nodes are more likely to present and embrace new ideas. The theory espouses that individual traits matter less than relationships between nodes in a network. SNA is most widely used in commercial organizations and only recently has been applied to health systems. In fact, in one systematic review, few studies could be found that used SNA (Chambers, Wilson, Thompson, & Harden, 2012); thus, its application in health care is limited.

Other change or transformation theories and translational models (such as the PARiHS [Promoting Action on Research Implementation in Health Services] framework; Kitson et al., 2008) can also help to describe the mechanisms whereby individuals, groups, and organizations adopt innovation. However, individual adoption is influenced by a number of interacting variables and much more empirical evidence is needed to better understand it.

Nonetheless, when reflecting on individual adoption from a leadership perspective, it is readily apparent that over time, individuals move from attitudes of indifference toward the new practice to increasingly more interest and ultimately to actively engaging with it, even, in some cases, trying to make it work better. At a system level, however, the adoption process is more complex and organizations, like individuals, can be classified as low, medium, or high adopters. Frambach and Schillewaert (2002) discussed two stages associated with system-level adoption: the organization's decision to pursue adoption and the staff's acceptance and initiation of their individual processes of accepting the innovation.

> Because individual adoption occurs in the context of an organization, the interaction between individual and organizational factors most likely affects the rate and comprehensiveness of adoption. Thus, even if the individual is motivated, ready, and capable, if the organization itself presents barriers, adoption may not be the result.

It is particularly challenging to promote change in routine practice when the decision to adopt is complicated by organizational factors such as a long-standing culture, deficient resources, and ineffective leadership. However, some drivers of adoption (facilitators) have been identified that can move organizations from medium or low adopters to high adopters. For example, organizational resources, training, positive social networks, and evidence of efficacy have been shown to be positively associated with adoption (Greenhalgh et al., 2004; Oldenburg & Glanz, 2008). In fact, in a synthesis paper, Wisdom et al. (2014) compared constructs related to organizational adoption of innovation and found several factors that favored adoption: positive sociopolitical external influences; leadership support and experience; research infrastructure; resources; positive social interactions (climate); easy-to-use innovations that were viewed as better than current practice, cost-effective, adaptable to the organization, and evidence-based; employees' positive attitudes toward change and other characteristics; frequent feedback; and system readiness for change. Contrarily, innovation adoption was limited in systems in which the innovation was perceived as complex, top-down hierarchical leadership situated in formal organizational structures was used, a poor climate persisted, innovation evidence was lacking, negative individual characteristics of employees persisted, lack of skills continued, and job tenure endured. Although this literature synthesis organized various frameworks, the relative lack of evidence available to clearly point out which factors facilitate system-level adoption was a major limitation.

TIPPING POINTS AND MILESTONES

Tipping Points

Over time, critical points in the evolving PPM integration lead to new and irreversible changes—these can be positive (manifested as progress) or negative (status quo). Often, it is a small detail, such as a certain nurse, or a particular unit, or a specified number of units, that get inspired by the model and can have the largest effect on the rest of the system. In Malcolm Gladwell's book, *The Tipping Point: How Little Things Can Make a Big Difference* (Gladwell, 2002), he likens tipping points to epidemics. In other words, in epidemics one or a few individuals become infected with contagious organisms and then transmit them in certain environments. Epidemics, then, are a function of a few people who transmit the organism or disease itself, and the environment in which it is operating. When an epidemic tips, it is jolted out of equilibrium, because of a change in one or all three of these areas.

When applied to an innovation, for example, Gladwell's law of a few (a tiny percentage of the people who do the most work), the stickiness factor (the degree to which a message [e.g., PPM] attaches and makes an impact), and the power of context (the situation or circumstances) strongly influences ongoing implementation and ultimate integration. Certain influential individuals whom Gladwell called the "mavens," are the recognized experts on a subject. Their adoption of a new innovation could influence colleagues who know them to consider adopting that innovation as well, but, on their own, these mavens are often so focused on their small world of expert knowledge that they fail to make the innovation real. "Connectors" are those who spread the word of the innovation to the broader world, linking influential people and ideas to create the interest and curiosity that attract early adopters like honey. Finally, the "salesmen" take the ideas spread by the connectors and persuade their acquaintances to actually try out an innovation. Like Rogers's (2003) Diffusion of Innovation Theory, Gladwell's underlying model explains that an innovation spreads rapidly when the right combination of these factors is present.

Identifying early who these few key people are (mavens, connectors, and salesmen), harnessing their energy, and relying on their knowledge and resources facilitate adoption. In terms of the stickiness factor, relatively simple changes in the PPM diagram or the presentation and structuring of information about a PPM can make a big difference. For example, including essential components of the underlying theory in the PPM image; using the model to explain existing policies and procedures; and applying small, focused skills-acquisition forums to present the model can force the model to "stick," pivoting (or tipping) the implementation toward advancement. Instead of a huge rollout, concentrating resources in a few key people and areas and helping to identify what is in it for the stakeholders, including how the change will impact their reality, may be more effective.

> By mobilizing the champions for change with the most influence, making incremental changes that stick, and establishing a positive context for change, the thresholds for innovating or trying something new may tip in the right direction.

Milestones

Milestones are noteworthy indicators or landmarks that signify progress throughout a project's life cycle. To warrant that designation, the marker must be of such significance that it exposes the nature of the progress in and of itself, even without any details relating to the specific, underlying work elements. For example, daily implementation of a PPM strategy is not a milestone, but having a sufficient number of such strategies in place across a system might be (see criteria for project milestones in Table 8.1).

Table 8.1 Key Criteria for Milestone Selection

1. The marker is important in and of itself relative to the overall execution of the project
2. If this landmark/breakthrough is not met on time, serious negative implications will transpire
3. The marker/event itself points to the project's success

> Project milestones set the stage to measure progress and can be used to manage the work effort and report meaningful status reports to stakeholders. Project milestones provide important signals regarding impact and value and suggest the plan's sustainability.

Uptake of innovation, or the evidence that adoption has occurred in a system, is necessary to validate the potential of a PPM to improve practice, positively impacting patient, nurse, and system outcomes, while also affirming the benefits of the organization's investment. After individuals process the PPM and adapt it to better fit the organization's needs (using local language and embedding it in familiar operations), its overall uptake can be observed.

> Typically, uptake of new behaviors is initially observed as feasibility (e.g., the practice is successfully carried out in the real world), it is satisfactory to those using it, it is deemed appropriate or suitable for a particular patient population, and is cost-effective (or has some other benefit). Actually using the new behaviors to improve practice is further evidence of its uptake.

For example, after practicing according to a particular PPM for a while, nurses on a unit might create a new policy grounded by the model, following the usual system processes for policy approval, and place the organizational logo on it. This approach matches other organizational policies, "institutionalizing" it so that staff accept it as the new norm. The extent to which the new policy is used (e.g., number of nurses using it, the units involved), awareness of and adherence to the new policy, and the expected consequences of it to patients, nurses, and systems (e.g., clinical outcomes, nurse satisfaction, resources used) is vital uptake evidence for health systems.

Determining uptake of a PPM by individuals, departments, and health systems contributes to a better understanding of the relative effectiveness of model components, the strategies that contribute to successful implementation, and provides important feedback and reinforcement necessary for engaging clinicians in new ways of practice. Of course, rapid feedback (requiring real-time data collection and analysis) may accelerate the desired change in practice. As evidence of uptake is made available, clinicians may be more likely to "see" the connection between PPM concepts and clinical practice, lending more credibility to the work.

WHEN VALUES BECOME REALITY: MEANINGFUL WORK

Because nursing work represents a huge investment of time among RNs, the meaning it provides is crucial to nurses' continued interest in, engagement with, and actual performance of the practice. *Meaningful* (2015) is defined as something that is significant, relevant, worthwhile, purposeful, and produces value. When experienced, it typically generates positive attitudes and feelings and may impact behavior. According to Steger, Dik, and Duffy (2012), meaningful work is dependent on both the individual and the organization. Individuals bring a sense of meaning and mission with them to the workplace through their individual characteristics, whereas organizations create meaningful (or meaningless) work environments. As Rosso and colleagues (2010) point out, meaningful work is often a subjective experience that what one does has significance. Furthermore, empirical research has shown that work frequently is an important source of meaning in life as a whole (Steger & Dik, 2010), suggesting that meaningful work may help people deepen their understanding of themselves and the world around them, facilitating their personal growth. Finally, the desire to make a positive impact on the greater good is consistently related to the experience of meaningful work (Grant, 2007), suggesting that work is most meaningful if it has a broader impact on others.

Lips-Wiersma and Wright (2012) identified four dimensions of meaningful work: developing the inner self, unity with others, service to others, and expressing full potential. Steger and Dik (2010), on the other hand, have provided a threefold definition of meaningful work that includes the degree to which people find their work to have significance and purpose, the contribution work makes to finding broader meaning in life, and the desire and means for one's work to make a positive contribution to the greater good. Both definitions provide a guide to the concept but Steger and Dik's definition seems more practical for the real world. This definition points to significant work as a contributor to one's overall life, and a force that generates a positive impact on society. As an integrated whole, these components of meaningful work can be expressed through a well-crafted PPM.

Professional practice models address the significance of nursing work by affirming important nursing values. In fact, the foundation for professional practice models is the organizational mission and articulated nursing values! Professional practice models also specify potential impact on others, namely, patients, nurses, and health systems. For example, many professional practice models allude to specific measurable outcomes of benefit (e.g., improved patient outcomes, more satisfied nurses).

The influence nursing work has on the broader meaning in life is much more personal, but nevertheless many nurses have voiced how their relationships with patients and families have positively influenced their lives (Duffy, 2013; Hunt, 2009). In short, the uptake of PPMs may provide nurses with the components of meaningful work that have been linked to work engagement and organizational commitment (Geldenhuys, Łaba, & Venter, 2014) as well as worker satisfaction, retention, and productivity (Brown et al., 2001; International Council of Nurses, 2007; Lieff, 2009). In fact, one group of researchers found that meaningfulness was the most significant determinant of work engagement (May, Gilson, & Harter, 2004).

> Creating the conditions for meaningful work in which nurses at all levels experience connection to the values that drove them to nursing in the first place and contribute to highly valued outcomes is a joint nurse–nurse leader responsibility.

Altering what nurses actually do and/or shaping the context within which nursing work is performed, including role redesign (Chapter 5), increasing employee involvement, improving obstacles from nurses' real work, and freeing them to perform their own work are examples of leader influences. Finally, by continuing to link the shared values undergirding the PPM to everyday work, leaders can facilitate a sense of integrated wholeness in which individuals, working supportively together at their full potential and in service to others, can make a large and positive contribution to others.

SUMMARY

Individual adoption of new behaviors was presented as a dynamic and complex process that involves a series of steps that occur dynamically in a certain context. Five conceptual frameworks were used to provide the foundation for understanding the individual adoption process: the transtheoretical model, SCT, Diffusion of Innovation, TPB, and SNA. At the system level, facilitators and barriers to adoption were identified. Tipping points and milestones were compared and important links to project progress were outlined. Validating that a PPM has indeed made the impact intended reflects the uptake of the model and is necessary to better understand the organization's investment. Finally, how a PPM provides the context for meaningful work with implications for nurse leaders was defended.

REFLECTIVE APPLICATIONS

For Students

1. Discuss how the work environment plays a role in individual adoption of new behaviors.
2. Describe the stages of change in the transtheoretical model. How can you use this to explain how you adopt new behaviors?
3. Discriminate among Rogers's five stages of adoption. Provide an example of each.
4. Describe a situation in which you adopted a new behavior. What did you do? What "tipped" you over to the new behavior? How did you know that uptake had occurred?
5. Explain how a large network of linked nodes can help embrace new ideas. How would a smaller network limit new ideas? Provide an example of each from your experience.
6. Explain how identifying early adopters can facilitate adoption in a health system. Have you seen this in your career? If yes, please explain.
7. List three drivers of adoption. What is leadership's role in applying such drivers?
8. Read Malcolm Gladwell's book, *The Tipping Point*. What is the main message? How could you use this in your future role?

For Clinical Nurses

1. Describe the significance of early adopters in integration of a PPM.
2. Analyze the PPM at your health system. Discuss its relative advantage, compatibility, complexity, "trialability," and observability. Be specific and provide examples. How could these characteristics be leveraged to foster individual adoption?
3. Name three barriers that exist in your institution that could slow down individual adoption of new practice behaviors. How do you know? What could you do to decrease their influence?
4. How often are you asked to consider adopting new practice behaviors? Be specific. What facilitators or drivers hasten your individual adoption? What are the latest examples as they relate to your department?
5. How does your health system facilitate the conditions for meaningful work? Be specific and provide examples.
6. Suggest three ideas that you could do to derive greater meaning in your work. How could you spread these ideas to coworkers?
7. What role does leadership play in facilitating uptake of new behaviors at your health system? What role do you play?

8. Name two milestones that you have used to judge the adoption of new behaviors. What were they? Did they work?

9. What methods would you advocate for creating an epidemic of new practice behaviors in your unit? Defend your answer.

For Nurse Leaders

1. Who in your organization are early adopters? Who are laggards? How do you know and what are their characteristics? Have you tapped them as a resource? Why is this significant?

2. How can Rogers's five stages of adoption be applied to integration of a PPM? Be specific. Who or what could help you with this?

3. Name three drivers and three barriers of adoption in your health system. How do these system attributes contribute to or detract from the innovation? How do you limit the barriers while applying the drivers? Name a large project in which you have used this approach. Did it work?

4. Explain how SNA could expose hidden relationships and collaborations in your system.

5. What is the "stickiness" factor? How could you use this to enhance implementation strategies? Can you identify someone in the organization whom you could work with on this?

6. Explain how meaningful work is tied to PPMs. How do you ensure meaningful work for nurses in your areas of responsibility? What signs would lead you to think that nurses already perceive their work as meaningful? Why? What can be done to increase the perception of meaningful work in your health system?

7. How do you identify milestones in large projects? Are they documented and reported? After reading this chapter, would you change your approach? Why or why not?

8. What tipping points have you experienced in your career that you could share with others?

9. List some markers that you could use to validate that "uptake" has occurred in PPM integration. Why did you select these? How would you disseminate them?

10. As a nurse leader, how do you ensure your own work is meaningful? What values is it tied to? How do you apply your work experiences to your wider life? What contributions from your work do you make to society? How could you leverage these characteristics to enhance your leadership?

11. Argue the pros and cons of your PPM. How do the theoretical frameworks in this chapter aid in this?

For Nurse Educators

1. How can undergraduate and graduate students best learn about individual adoption?
2. What learning strategies will you use to help students understand the many theoretical notions of individual adoption? How will you ensure that the concepts are tied to the real world?
3. Develop a teaching strategy for helping nurse leaders better examine the concept of meaningful work. How will you evaluate this?
4. How could you begin to help undergraduate nursing students examine the meaning in their work? What concepts would you use? How would you evaluate it?
5. How could you help fellow faculty members better teach the concept of meaningful work? What teaching practices would you recommend?
6. How would you guide students at all levels to examine characteristics of PPMs that might inform their selection in the work environment? What conceptual framework would you use? Why?
7. What methods do you think would help students at all levels to understand the concept uptake?
8. Read Malcolm Gladwell's book, *The Tipping Point*. How could you use its message to encourage adoption of new curricular evaluation methods? Provide examples.

LEARNING FROM THE FIELD: INDIVIDUAL ADOPTION OF THE QUALITY-CARING MODEL©

When I was first introduced to the Quality-Caring Model (Duffy, 2009) as the selected practice modality for Novant Health Prince William Medical Center, I was very intrigued. This model is completely encompassing to all aspects of the role of the nurse in relation to taking care of patients. For me, I find I am able to provide remarkable care following this theoretical framework.

I recently had the pleasure of caring for a patient, R. S., who was a 61-year-old female admitted postoperatively after a colectomy and colostomy placement. During my time caring for R. S., I was able to apply many aspects of the Quality-Caring Model. R. S. was experiencing a few medical complications in addition to major body and lifestyle changes. Sensing that R. S. was scared and nervous about her condition and recovery, I used the caring factor of attentive reassurance to first notice her response and then console and encourage her by pointing out that she was in a stable condition and would soon begin feeling stronger. Using mutual problem solving, I took the necessary time to show and explain the colostomy to R. S. and her husband, answering any questions or concerns they verbalized, all the while allowing them to engage in the process. On hearing that R. S. had a difficult time sleeping the night before and using the caring factor of healing environment, I made sure R. S. had a quiet atmosphere with limited interruptions in order to promote rest the next day. This also involved providing pain and antinausea medications proactively so as not to disturb her needed rest.

When R. S. began to feel a little better, I advocated for an increase in her diet to clear liquids. This allowed her basic human needs, such as thirst and appetite, to be satisfied. As she continued to progress, I discussed the remaining plan of care with R. S. and her husband, codeveloped a timeline for activities of daily living, such as bathing and ambulating, and began discharge plans. Using this model reminds me of the important nursing emphasis on patients and families (versus those nonrelational aspects of the work), how nursing influences patient outcomes, and above all, contributes to helping me remember the important work I do.

Shauna Bendix

REFERENCES

Ajzen, I. (1985). From intentions to actions: A theory of planned behavior. In J. Kuhl & J. Beckmann (Eds.), *Action control: From cognition to behavior* (pp. 11–39). New York, NY: Springer-Verlag.

Ajzen, I. (1991). The theory of planned behavior. *Organization Behavior and Human Decision Processes, 50,* 170–211.

Andrews, V., Tonkin, E., Lancastle, D., & Kirk, M. (2014). Identifying the characteristics of nurse opinion leaders to aid the integration of genetics in nursing practice. *Journal of Advanced Nursing, 70*(11), 2598–2611.

Bandura, A. (1969). *Principles of behavior modification.* New York, NY: Holt, Rinehart, and Wilson.

Brown, A., Kitchell, M., O'Neill, T., Lockliear, J., Vosler, A., Kubek, D., & Dale, L. (2001). Identifying meaning and perceived level of satisfaction within the context of work. *Work, 16,* 219–226.

Chambers, D., Wilson, P., Thompson, C., & Harden, M. (2012). Social network analysis in healthcare settings: A systematic scoping review. *PLoS one, 7*(8), e41911.

Clarke, R. (1996). *A primer in diffusion of innovations theory.* Retrieved February 2, 2015, from http://www.anu.edu.au/people/Roger. Clarke/SOS/InnDiff.html

Duffy, J. (2009). *Quality caring in nursing: Apply theory to clinical practice, education and leadership*. New York, NY: Springer Publishing Company.

Duffy, J. R. (2013). *Quality caring in nursing and health systems: Implications for clinical practice, education, and leadership*. New York, NY: Springer Publishing Company.

Frambach, R. T., & Schillewaert, N. (2002). Organizational innovation adoption: A multi-level framework of determinants and opportunities for future research. *Journal of Business Research*, 55(2), 163–176.

Geldenhuys, M., Łaba, K., & Venter, C. M. (2014). Meaningful work, work engagement and organisational commitment. *South African Journal of Industrial Psychology*, 40(1), 10. doi:10.4102/sajip.v40i1.1098

Gladwell, M. (2002). *The tipping point: How little things can make a big difference*. New York, NY: Little, Brown.

Grant, A. (2007). Relational job design and the motivation to make a prosocial difference. *Academy of Management Review*, 32(2), 393–417.

Greenhalgh, T., Robert, G., MacFarlane, F., Bate, P., & Kyriakidou, O. (2004). Diffusion of innovation in service organizations: Systematic review and recommendations. *Milbank Quarterly*, 82(4), 581–629.

Hunt, R. J. (2009, November). *Meaningful moments in public health nursing*. Paper presented at the American Public Health Association, Philadelphia, PA.

International Council of Nurses (ICN). (2007). *Positive practice environments*. Geneva, Switzerland: Author.

Kitson, A. L., Rycroft-Malone, J., Harvey, G., McCormack, B., Seers, K., & Titchen, A. (2008). Evaluating the successful implementation of evidence into practice using the PARiHS framework: Theoretical and practical challenges. *Implementation Science*, 3, 1.

Lieff, S. J. (2009). The missing link in academic career planning and development: Pursuit of meaningful and aligned work. *Academic Medicine*, 84, 1383–1388.

Lips-Wiersma, M., & Wright, S. (2012). Measuring the meaning of meaningful work: Development and validation of the Comprehensive Meaningful Work Scale (CMWS). *Group & Organization Management*, 37(5), 655–685.

May, D. R., Gilson, R. L., & Harter, L. M. (2004). The psychological conditions of meaningfulness, safety and availability and the engagement of the human spirit at work. *Journal of Occupational and Organizational Psychology*, 77, 11–37.

Meaningful. (2015). Retrieved February 2, 2015 from http://dictionary.reference.com/browse/meaningful

Oldenburg, B., & Glanz, K. (2008). Diffusion of innovations. In K. Glanz, B. K. Rimer, & K. Viswanath (Eds.), *Health behavior and health education* (4th ed., pp. 313–333). San Francisco, CA: Jossey-Bass.

Prochaska, J. O., & DiClemente, C. (1983). Stages and processes of self-change in smoking: Toward an integrative model of change. *Journal of Consulting and Clinical Psychology*, 5, 390–395.

Prochaska, J. O., DiClemente, C. C., & Norcross, J. C. (1992). In search of how people change: Applications to addictive behaviors. *American Psychologist, 47*(9), 1102–1112.

Rogers, E. M. (1962). *Diffusion of innovations* (1st ed.). New York, NY: Free Press.

Rogers, E. M. (1995). *Diffusion of innovations* (4th ed.). New York, NY: Free Press.

Rogers, E. M. (2003). *Diffusion of innovations* (5th ed.). New York, NY: Free Press.

Rosso, B. B., Dekas, K. H., & Wrzesmoewsli, A. (2010). On the meaning of work: A theoretical integration and review. *Research in Organizational Behavior, 30*(12), 91–127.

Steger, M. F., & Dik, B. J. (2010). Work as meaning. In P. A. Linley, S. Harrington, & N. Page (Eds.), *Oxford handbook of positive psychology and work* (pp. 131–142). Oxford, UK: Oxford University Press.

Steger, M. F., Dik, B. J., & Duffy, R. D. (2012). Measuring meaningful work: The work and meaning inventory. *Journal of Career Assessment, 20,* 322–337.

Wasserman, S., & Faust, K. (1994). *Social network analysis: Methods and applications.* Cambridge, UK: Cambridge University Press.

Wisdom, J. P., Chor, K. H. B, Hoagwood, K. E., & Horwitz, S. M. (2014). Innovation adoption: A review of theories and constructs. *Administrative Policy in Mental Health, 41,* 480–502.

CHAPTER 9

Values and Behaviors Associated With Exemplary Professional Practice: Enculturation

Socialization, resocialization, enculturation, onboarding, talent development, competencies

By the end of this chapter, readers will be able to:

1. Define the terms *socialization*, *resocialization*, and *enculturation* related to professional nurse work
2. Describe the term *cultural "fit"*
3. Evaluate how hiring practices, onboarding, and talent development contribute to enculturation
4. Differentiate between generic and technical competencies
5. Apply principles of accountability related to a professional practice model (PPM)
6. Analyze evidence for successful PPM enculturation

HEALTH SYSTEM ENCULTURATION

In today's global workforce, nurses frequently change employment while, at the same time, health systems busily modify their traditions in response to external reimbursement/accreditation forces and internal practice improvement. The transferability of nurses' clinical skills to new or altered health systems is implied, but the cultural specificity of these skills can often be a barrier to successful professional assimilation (Neiterman & Bourgeault, 2015). In fact, studies of new nurse socialization practices emphasize how nursing's ethos of caring can be lost to one of competence during the process as beginners transition from student to RN (Mackintosh, 2006; Price, 2009).

Although the majority of nurse socialization literature focuses on those new to the profession, the concept of resocialization is beginning to emerge in terms of appreciating that professional practice is embedded in the wider cultural and political ideologies of health systems. As such, employees often must unlearn, relearn, and acquire relevant system-specific language, norms, and practices. Thus, nursing knowledge and skill is not sufficient for individual career and organizational success. Rather, ongoing individual learning and recurrent modifications to professional nurse work and accommodation to the professional identity of health systems are necessary.

Socializing or resocializing nurses to the underlying values, norms, expectations, and acceptable behaviors (culture) of a health system is typically accomplished through orientation and/or educational programs, which can last anywhere from 2 hours to several weeks (depending on the system and the employee). Yet, to be successful (in terms of job performance and proficiency), nurses not only need to understand the work, but also require an understanding of institutional history, stories, and legends; goals and politics; how decisions are made; the language required to communicate effectively; important symbols and artifacts; values and daily work behaviors necessary to "fit" in, and acquire a sense of belonging (Chao, O'Leary-Kelly, Wolf, Klein, & Gardner, 1994).

The concept of enculturation is used to describe this dynamic process of learning, experiencing, and assimilating system values, expectations, and obligations, and how nursing occurs, including its proper behaviors, language, and interactions.

Enculturation is a socialization process by which employees adjust to, and eventually become part of, the unique culture of their health system (Tutlas, 2011). This unique culture is often made up of unspoken and unwritten rules for working together. In fact, E. Adamson Hoebel (1949), a distinguished anthropologist, noted that enculturation is both a conscious and an unconscious conditioning process whereby a person achieves competence in his or her culture and internalizes it. If successful, enculturation provides a clearer understanding of the complexities of the system and results in competence in the language, values, and rituals of the culture—in essence it ensures a "fit" between the system and the employee. As expected, employees who are good cultural fits work well in a health system, whereas those who fail to fit in the environment either become marginalized and unsuccessful or leave to find a more congruent work environment.

In terms of professional practice models (PPMs), enculturation assumes that nurses acquire the knowledge, skills, and attitudes associated with the model, are responsive to it, and are motivated to behave according to its tenets. In other words, they acquire the competence to practice it, are motivated to continuously improve their practice, reflect on how the PPM informs the larger discipline of nursing, and develop a professional identity that aligns with the model.

> Inspiring employees to deliver on the professional practice model is a leadership responsibility that ensures nursing work is performed in accordance with a health system's unique ethos (i.e., "the way we practice nursing here").

ALIGNMENT WITH THE PROFESSIONAL PRACTICE MODEL

> Because the professional practice model essentially brands the practice of nursing for a health system, it clarifies for any nurse what is "appropriate practice" versus what is "inappropriate practice." In doing so, it becomes easier to make the right clinical decisions.

Because nursing practice often carries over or influences other health professionals' practice, the whole health system will eventually have a lens that enables smart and appropriate clinical decisions based on the selected PPM. Building such a culture is not a short-term activity or announcement; rather, it is a genuine and ongoing commitment to the organization's PPM, resulting in employees who are consistently living the model both inside and outside the system on a daily basis.

Employees must grasp the meaning of the professional practice model and how it translates into observable, actionable behaviors that can positively impact the entire system.

Typically, employees move through three stages: from awareness of the model to advocating for it (based on how well leadership is committed at the highest levels, the particular strategies and evaluation feedback that was implemented [Chapters 5 and 6], and ongoing enthusiasm about how the model is spread; Figure 9.1). In Figure 9.1, new employees begin their integration to the PPM during the onboarding process during which the conceptual foundation is laid. Over time and with specific strategies, they begin to emotionally attach to the model, eventually accepting it and, finally, they begin to identify with the model, using and promoting it daily. This is a long-term process that unravels over many months, sometimes years. New employees must modify their professional identity enough to meet the standards of professional practice at a specific health system, oftentimes balancing the need to present themselves as competent while at the same time ascertaining how they can adjust their behavior in order to fit in. Groups of nurses (departments) who eventually become deeply aligned with the PPM maximize its strength and contribute to a more lively professionally based culture. For example, living a PPM:

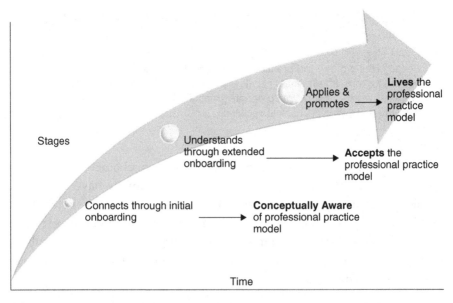

Figure 9.1 Progression of professional practice model translation.

- Provides a daily tangible reason for ongoing practice improvement
- Contributes to a level of pride tied to fulfilling the model's promises
- May facilitate recruitment and retention
- Confirms the focus of nursing practice
- Generates positive energy necessary for engagement
- Shows employees how they fit into the health system's values and priorities

Alignment with the PPM starts with selecting the right employees.

Hiring Practices and the Professional Practice Model

Hiring nurses based on skill competency alone is not the best approach for enculturating a PPM.

Rather, finding superior talent (talent acquisition) that fits the workplace culture requires finding candidates who have the potential for the same key behaviors that are required to practice the selected professional practice model. The candidate whose values, beliefs, outlook, and behavior are congruent with the professional practice model *and* those existing within the current system is mostly likely to be a good cultural fit for the organization.

Of course, this means that nursing and human resources departments must be on the same page regarding candidate selection, and the human resources staff must understand the PPM enough that successful hiring (and future enculturation) is accomplished. Searching for candidates who are knowledgeable about nursing as a profession, including its significance, are energetic and interpersonally skilled, committed, passionate, patient centered, and who are comfortable taking risks is essential (Table 9.1).

Prior to or during integration of a PPM, exploring the health system's talent acquisition program, including the processes of finding, assessing, and eventually hiring nurses who meet the organizations' requirements for practice, is beneficial. For example, being aware of schools of nursing or other health systems that have similar values and attitudes about nursing is an important strategy. This may require searching others' websites, seeking out and making connections with educational program directors, and speaking with potential candidates at specific professional conferences. Inquiring of recent hires how the recruiting process might be improved may yield important information. Ensuring that the PPM is prominently positioned on the job

Table 9.1 Culturally Congruent Candidate Characteristics

Knowledge	Passion	Risk Taker	Energy	Patient Centered	Commitment
Demonstrates understanding of professional nursing	Excited by opportunity	Exposes oneself	Engages in conversations	Relates to patients as mutual partners	Dedicated to lifelong learning
States the significance of nursing	Attracted by clinical unit	Sees possibilities	Greets others warmly	Demonstrates accountability for patient well-being	Can execute a long-term project
Comprehends the responsibilities associated with professional nursing	Enthusiastic about professional practice model	Shows innovativeness	Is animated during interview	States being with patients and families as meaningful	Sees oneself in nursing in 10 years

description so that potential employees can judge their likely fit when they first examine the requirements for working at a specific health system is valuable. Tailoring the interview for the specific setting and critical role competencies is important, that is, expressing the organization's mission and nursing values, walking potential employees through a clinical unit and describing the experiences they will encounter should they be hired, observing their interactions with presently employed nurses, and asking the candidates questions about their potential suitability generates valuable information. In some cases, assessment tools are available for evaluating potential employee values and competencies and can be used again after hire to design an appropriate onboarding program. Asking open-ended, behavior-based questions on interview, eliciting responses that might forecast future performance, also called behavioral interviewing (Clifford, 2006; Huffcutt, Van Iddekinge, & Roth, 2011), facilitates successful hires. Some examples include:

- Can you tell me about a situation that was uncomfortable (risky) for you? What happened? What did you do? How do you feel about it now?
- Tell us what your plans are 10 years from now? What will occupy your time? Can you provide an example?
- What significance do you think nursing makes in the lives of patients? Families? Other health professionals? Why?

- Can you provide an example of a time when you believe you were practicing "professional" nursing? How do you know? What were the patient's responses?
- Can you tell us about a time when you felt very strongly about a patient or a patient situation. What was the end result? What steps did you take to make this happen?

Finally, despite the fact that letters of reference, background checks, and transcripts are considered essential hiring practices, this author has witnessed several scenarios of employees being hired without such validating information. Consider the following case:

> A large system had a vacancy posted for a job that required a master's degree and some work experience related to the specific position. The hiring practices at the system required a search committee made up of peers. Thus, the search committee conducted a series of interviews with potential candidates, per policy. A particular candidate described his or her prior work experience, stating verbally and in writing that graduate work was done at a specific university. The search committee concluded this person was a good candidate and developed a recommendation for hire. It is not the routine practice of the human resources department at this system to solicit reference letters or transcripts; rather they rely on search committee recommendations. The recommended individual was hired and a year later, after some negative work evaluations, it was discovered that the individual never *completed* the required graduate degree. Upon questioning, the search committee revealed they never solicited transcripts—rather, they "assumed the human resources department did that." The individual remains in the position, although he/she is not able to successfully execute its requirements.

How often do hiring practices such as this result in a poor fit between the organization's needs and the employee's competencies and values?

Background checks provide general character information that does not reflect the candidate's job performance, but does give an overall picture of the candidate's behavior. Reference checks and official transcripts, however, are much more focused, and can garner important information that can facilitate the system's success in hiring.

Onboarding

Onboarding is "the process of acquiring, accommodating, assimilating, and accelerating new team members" (Bradt & Vonnegut, 2009, p. 3). Stated another way, "onboarding is the process of helping new hires adjust to social and performance aspects of their new jobs quickly and smoothly" (Bauer, 2010, p. 1). Effective onboarding drives employee productivity, accelerates the delivery of results, and improves retention (Bradt & Vonnegut, 2009). It can be a culture-shaping process that gives a competitive advantage to one health system over another, provided it is conducted for success. Unfortunately, only about 20% of organizations achieve this level of onboarding, creating less than desirable results (reduced manager and hourly worker assimilation and retention; Bauer, 2010; Hall, 2013). And, to decrease costs of onboarding, many health systems have shortened the process.

Overwhelming new employees with large amounts of information in a short period of time may be counterproductive, leading to failure of the process. Rather, an extended onboarding process that accommodates employees' needs not just for compliance, but for better understanding of the health system itself (history, values, mission, politics), how to interact with others in the system, competencies required for the particular role, the language associated with the PPM, and important connections to others is recommended. Some examples of such successful onboarding processes include:

- Question-and-answer time with the chief operating officer or another similar executive-level administrator who demonstrates commitment to the PPM
- An overview of the system's culture and future goals
- A breakdown of the various roles within the organization, including associated responsibilities
- An outline of potential career paths for employees
- A diagram of the new employee's workplace connections
- Welcoming attitude beginning on the first day
- Exposure of new employees to various relevant departments
- An effective preceptor, mentor, or transition coach strategy in which new hires are paired with seasoned employees over time
- Extracurricular bonding opportunities such as sports events, dinners, or service projects

Noticeably absent from the preceding list are specific nursing skills; rather, factors that are specific to creating a lasting bond between a new employee and the health system are dominant. "Research has established that new employees who feel connected and accepted by their new colleagues have less initial anxiety upon entering the new organization" (Bauer, 2013, p. 5). To ensure a successful cultural fit, new employees need information and experiences that help them learn how "to be" in the health system. Such learning facilitates assimilation of values, appropriate behaviors, and system interaction norms. A written onboarding plan with associated training, coaching, precepting, frequent feedback, participatory approaches delivered consistently over time, and evaluations of important employee milestones is essential. As previously indicated, this process is most successful when the human resource and nursing departments work together for the good of the employee to consciously shape a work culture that ensures the success of the PPM. Outcomes from successful onboarding include employee self-efficacy, role clarity, social integration, and knowledge of the culture in the short term and then, optimistically, job satisfaction and organizational commitment in the long term (Bauer, 2010).

Talent Development

Talent (or aptitude) is a concept that refers to some exemplary characteristic that certain people possess (Garavan, Carbery, & Rock, 2012). The concept can be defined at three levels: individual, group, and organizational. Individually, it is described as a unique, exceptional, outstanding ability or skills in a certain area or topic. It may also refer to a person who is creative, innovative, and achieves superior results, for example, the athlete or musician who is deemed quite talented. At the group level, the talent of one individual is blended in among several individuals, whereas at the organizational level, collective employee talent is considered essential to achieving the overall aspirations of the system. In this case, organizational "talent" can be viewed as referring to a pool of employees (nurses and those who support them) who possess unique capacities (or have the potential to develop them) that facilitate nursing work as defined by the selected PPM.

Health systems define talent specific to their organizations; thus, it is a dynamic concept that changes over time based on organizational goals. As such, health systems bear the burden of talent development, making it an expensive and time-consuming endeavor. Talent development "focuses on the planning, selection and implementation of developmental strategies for the entire talent pool to ensure that the organization has both the current and future supply of talent to meet strategic objectives" (Jamka, 2011, p. 65). Thus, talent development is a focused, evolving process that requires highly engaged professionals who work in tandem with employees to ensure up-to-date health system capacity.

Talent emerges progressively from the transformation of individual aptitudes (or raw material) to systematically developed skills that are catalyzed by intrapersonal and environmental forces (Gagné, 2000). The process of talent development manifests as systematic learning followed by practicing. The higher the level of talent sought, the more intensive is the process required. In a practice-oriented profession such as nursing, the critical component of practice or experiential application cannot be overstated. Role models become highly influential to new employees in this process as do the relationships developed with other health care professionals. Emerging talent is manifested as "credible individuals who consistently deliver strong results; master new types of expertise quickly, recognize the importance of behavior, relentlessly focus on learning, have an entrepreneurial spirit with the capacity to take risks" (Micheals, Handfield-Jones, & Axelrod, 2001, p. 111). Such individuals exude competence, accountability, and engagement.

Competencies Required for Professional Practice

Competencies are the skills and personal characteristics required for superior performance (Workitect, 2012). They focus on specific behaviors that can be grouped into two domains: generic and technical. Generic competencies are highly contextual (Dierdorff, Rubin, & Morgeson, 2009) and include role, social, and physical dimensions. For example, role competencies focus on the informational and structural features of the professional role, as well as accountability and autonomy (Johns, 2006). The social dimension focuses on interpersonal aspects of the role such as communication, conflict, the degree of interdependence, and density of human interaction. Physical context focuses on issues, such as the working conditions like degree of risk, hazard, noise, and so on, which influence work performance and behavior. Unlike technical competence, generic competencies provide more significant developmental challenges.

Generic competencies tend to be holistic, to overlap, and interweave (Capaldo, Landoli, & Zollo, 2006), and they are intrinsically tied to personal characteristics such as self-confidence, motivation, and interpersonal skills. Talented employees are expected to display generic competencies that meet the demands of a unique and continually changing work environment, which requires flexibility of process (Garazonik, Nethersell, & Spreier, 2006).

One approach to generic competency identification is to use competency maps that help identify key core competencies for a health system that can be used to guide employee development, provide a common language, and assess attainment (Isrealite, 2010). These maps are typically standardized across all units of a health system with established domains used to identify both individual and business unit development needs. For example, domains for generic competencies might include health system mission, goals, strategic plan, and role in community; role and identity of health system leadership; general communication mechanisms; the performance evaluation and advancement processes; appreciating diversity; dress and behavior codes. Mixed reviews on competency maps are apparent in the literature without good empirical evidence of their long-term value.

Technical competencies, on the other hand, include the knowledge, skills, and attitudes required for a specific task, that is, professional nursing. In this case, such competencies are derived from professional standards, state nurse practice acts, and the PPM. Examples of nursing-specific competency domains might include observation and communication (obtain accurate and pertinent information from patients, e.g., comprehensive assessment), motor (perform certain procedures), cognitive (interpret patient information, prioritize patient needs, retrieve and critically appraise research to determine the best available research evidence, develop plans of care), and communication (accurately convey information to health team members).

Within a professional practice model, however, competencies related to the behavioral translation of model concepts are vital. Over time and with knowledge followed by practice, employees will develop competency in the practice (as defined by the system's unique professional practice model) and its associated values, language, and rituals, and will evolve a professional identity that brings the model to life.

Accountability and Engagement

Accountability underpins professional nursing practice and refers to accepting responsibility for consistently doing the right thing. Because accountability is foundational to *professional* nursing practice, adhering to a particular *professional* practice model implies an obligation to practice congruently using the model while being answerable to oneself and others (with possible consequences) if the particular form of practice is not followed. It also confers ownership; that is, having power or control over the professional practice of nursing.

> Thus, the commitment to a professional practice model suggests a compelling
> duty to conform to its principles and a willingness to reflect on and continuously
> improve the practice.

As an organized body of nurses, this commitment to common ways of practicing and ongoing improvement in a health system ensures that clinical decisions and practice improvements are guided by a unifying framework (versus individual preference) and infers that situations in which such practice is not occurring are corrected.

> Such accountability is shared between nurses and nurse leaders and further
> advanced when both participants work together to meet the expectations
> of the professional practice model. Together, nurses and nurse leaders must
> examine the incentives and consequences of prolonging existing practice in
> spite of the commitment to a given professional practice model.

For example, nurses must ask themselves whether there is any evidence that current practice is of benefit to patients or the organization (versus themselves). Or, they could examine the existing evidence for benefits of the chosen PPM to garner support for its responsible delivery. Nurse leaders must remember their ethical responsibility for professional practice environments and facilitate a cohesive group of nurses who demonstrate accountability for the professional practice (as defined by the model) by expecting its consistent use and ensuring reasonable incentives, reporting mechanisms, and consequences are upheld to facilitate such practice.

> Working together, nurses and nurse leaders can promote accountability for
> the delivery of professional nursing practice by clarifying professional role
> responsibilities (and reviewing them often), providing guidance regarding how
> the professional practice model should be operationalized (with follow-up
> support) and delineating expectations for performance, while holding each
> other accountable for behavior vis-à-vis the professional practice model. In
> doing so, a culture of accountability regarding how nursing is practiced in an
> organization is fostered that specifies the basis for personal accountability and
> patients' ongoing trust.

It is within such a culture that nurse engagement may flourish.

Schaufeli and colleagues (2002) defined work engagement as "a positive, fulfilling, and work-related state of mind that is characterized by vigor, dedication, and absorption" (p. 465). Although work engagement in various disciplines has been associated with positive organizational outcomes (Keydo, 2014), work engagement in nursing practice is problematic. According to the Advisory Board Company (2014) of hospital-based nurses in the United States, 7.4% of front-line nurses remain disengaged and they lag behind other health professionals. In their report, *A Data Driven Approach to Nurse Engagement: Key Insights and Best Practices from the Experts* (Advisory Board Company, 2014), the authors pointed to unclear linkages between leaders' actions and the mission; not feeling valued, with lack of respect for individual contributions; lack of help with stress and burnout; limited promotion opportunities; training and development; and little recognition as impediments to nurse engagement.

In an environment committed to a PPM, the resultant application of meaningful work (Chapter 8) in which nursing values and practice are congruent, may expedite nurse engagement (Vinje & Mittelmark, 2008). Because work engagement is embedded in daily nursing practice, nurses who identify with and embody a PPM (i.e., exemplify the model in practice) recognize that nursing care is more than a set of tasks and procedures and autonomously combine their perceptions and relationships with patients and families with instrumental aspects of care to inform their practice. Over time, as groups of nurses in a health system fully embody the PPM, the resultant culture of accountability that is generated perpetuates work engagement. In other words, a snowball effect may occur that drives further work engagement and may mediate important patient, employee, and system outcomes.

It is reasonable to suggest that delivering care in accordance with a PPM links nursing values with practice and thus influences work engagement, although empirical evidence is needed to substantiate this. Nurse leaders who clearly link their actions with the PPM, value and recognize the associated practice behaviors demonstrated by nurses, and provide support to uphold the model may influence physically involved, cognitively vigilant, and emotionally connected nurses, as in Kahn's (1990) definition of engaged employees.

LIVING THE PROFESSIONAL PRACTICE MODEL

As groups of nurses acquire the values, expected behaviors, and local knowledge needed to operationalize the professional practice model, a living representation of the model expresses itself, inviting examination, improvement, and dissemination.

However, in most health systems, a tension exists between new employees (or those requiring resocialization) and the expected institutional culture. For example, a nurse who is a team player and who appreciates coworker input and collaboration with other health professionals is more likely to "fit in" to a health system that chose a PPM in which teamwork is considered integral to good practice. Contrarily, an employee who is a loner may not find a good cultural fit in that same team-oriented workplace.

Because employees generally want to please, they often perform the required behaviors but may do so in a phony manner. In nursing, this can be especially problematic, given the close relationship nurses have with patients and families. The challenge then for nursing leaders is not to force conformity to a PPM, but rather to hire those with similar values and expectations and/or to identify employees' strengths and use them to frame employees' roles as opportunities to use their unique strengths and perspectives at work, thereby bringing more of their authentic best selves to the practice (Seligman, Steen, Park, & Peterson, 2005). Such an approach may buffer the threat many newcomers experience, allowing them to authentically live the PPM and more easily fit into the created culture (Cable, Gino, & Staats, 2013).

Successful enculturation, resulting in nurses (including nurse leaders) who are excited and proud of their work, makes the PPM come alive through the nurses' behaviors and attitudes. Evidence of such enculturation can be seen in how people relate to one another, specific practice examples, leadership actions, and organizational documents.

For example, the PPM may be reflected in the nursing strategic plan, various policy statements, and procedural instructions that reflect and promote the PPM, and the defined patient care delivery system will be well aligned with the stated PPM. Furthermore, hiring decisions are made in light of the cultural "fit" with the PPM, job descriptions include performance expectations consistent with the particular model, and the system for performance appraisal includes components of the PPM.

In terms of the environment, unit artifacts are welcoming, informative, and consistent with the PPM, and there is evidence of PPM language in the medical record. Finally, when observing professional behaviors, employees show confidence in their ability to perform according to the PPM, use the model in practice such as in care planning and documentation (Table 9.2), can describe features of the model, are engaged in improving practice, and demonstrate accountability for the model by consistently ensuring model-guided professional attitudes and behaviors.

Overall, enculturated PPMs are evidenced by cultural norms (the "right way" to be and practice nursing in a health system) as expressed by employee behaviors, use of model language, artifacts and rituals, values, role specificity, and interactions.

Employees' ability to "absorb" these intangibles is a goal of most health systems However, serious difficulties remain that challenge nurse leaders. For example, it is not known what specific experiences, exposures, and challenges nurses need in order to emerge as living examples of a specific PPM or how a health system manages to provide a cost-efficient talent development program that bridges the gap between model concepts and practice. It is also not known what proportion of talent development is system versus individually directed or the time frame required to develop system-wide talent such that a specific way of practicing nursing is consistently performed at the highest level. In addition, the combination of human resources and nursing professionals that best contribute to talent development and the appropriateness and sequencing of competency maps for effective enculturation are also not well understood. Thus, nurse leaders are often working without a good evidence base. Although much work remains to be done, preliminary and anecdotal evidence is guiding the way forward.

SUMMARY

In this chapter, enculturation, in terms of translating profession practice model concepts into tangible clinical practices and norms of behavior, was described. The notion of professional practice embedded in the wider cultural norms of a health system, including associated unlearning, relearning, experiencing, and assimilating "how nursing occurs" was explored. Cultural "fit," a term that assumes nurses absorb the knowledge, skills, and values associated with a PPM and become competent practicing that way and are thereby willing to improve the practice, was presented. Employees' movement through various stages as they learn to grasp the meaning of the PPM was depicted and explained. Furthermore, as groups of nurses become deeply aligned with the model, a more lively professionally based culture begins to unfold.

Hiring and onboarding nurses who "fit" the designated practice culture is a human resource strategy that may facilitate more effective and efficient enculturation. Various interviewing techniques and onboarding strategies were offered with emphasis on ensuring the assimilation of appropriate system values, behaviors, and interactions. Ongoing talent development, a

Table 9.2 Evidence of a Professional Practice Model "Living" in Nursing Practice

Model Component	Nursing Process			EHR Documentation
	Assessment	Possible Nursing Diagnoses	Plan	Evaluation	Documentation
Caring Factor					
Mutual problem solving	Assess health readiness and preferred learning style	Knowledge deficit	1. Engage patient/family in dialog about illness	Patient expresses positive learning experiences	Observations of patients' behaviors
	Determine problem-solving style	Decisional conflict	2. Reframe health problems to allow for greater possible alternatives	Patient expresses increased ability to cope with illness	Teaching provided, including learning approach and responses
	Assess knowledge about illness and required treatment plan	Ineffective self-management	3. Facilitate learning through goal setting	Patient utilizes appropriate resources	Discussion with patients
	Assess coping ability	Ineffective coping	4. Tailor learning based on developmental and health literacy levels	Patient reports increased ability to meet demands of daily living	
		Ineffective role performance	5. Brainstorm together, ask open-ended questions, mutually explore how others deal with similar health problems	Patient identifies lifestyle changes, specific health strategies, and treatment regimens that will improve illness or ability to cope with illness	
		Nonadherence	6. Include patient in rounds and shift reports	Patient accepts the need to adjust lifestyle	
			7. Discuss necessary lifestyle changes	Patient makes informed choices related to health problems	
			8. Encourage two-way communication	Patient describes at least three basic concepts about his or her disease	
			9. Solicit feedback from patients	Patient states at least four strategies to improve self-care or improve ADLs	
			10. Accept and experiment with patients' ideas	Patient actively participates in learning opportunities	
				Increased knowledge	

ADL, activities of daily living; EHR, electronic health records.

focused, dynamic process that includes learning followed by practice, was described. Generic and technical competencies were compared and experiential learning was promoted. Accountability, as a shared process between nurses and nurse leaders, was advocated with both "owning" the responsibility for ensuring appropriate professional practice. Evidence of PPM enculturation in terms of specific practice behaviors, organizational procedures, and contextual artifacts was highlighted. Finally, continuing issues related to successful enculturation were emphasized pointing to the need for ongoing research.

REFLECTIVE APPLICATIONS

For Students

1. Differentiate among the terms *socialization, resocialization,* and *enculturation* as they pertain to nurses in a health system.
2. Think about the term *enculturation.* How important do you think it is to acquire the appropriate "norms of behavior" in a health system in order to "fit" in? How might enculturation affect your career?
3. How does a good cultural "fit" facilitate delivery of a PPM?
4. Examine Table 9.1. Provide a practice example from each of the three stages that represents that particular stage of progression.
5. Reflect on the statement "hiring nurses based on skill competency alone is not the best approach for enculturating a PPM" (p. 193). What are your thoughts about this? Have you seen examples of this in your clinical courses? If yes, please explain.
6. Examine Table 9.1. Evaluate yourself for each of the categories. How do you fare? What can you do to improve in specific categories?
7. Discuss how you can best prepare for interviewing in a health system.
8. What should you look for in a potential hiring situation regarding a health system's onboarding program? What about the talent development process? What questions could you ask during the interview that might elicit information about these programs?
9. Develop a competency map for generic and technical nursing competencies. Include three competencies for each category.
10. Provide an example of how you would ensure accountability for a PPM during a situation you witnessed in which a peer did not practice in accordance with it. How would you work together with the nurse leader to ensure accountability?
11. Explain how living a PPM may engender a sense of pride in your chosen profession.

For Clinical Nurses

1. Describe the significance of "cultural fit" in terms of enculturating a PPM.
2. Analyze the PPM at your health system. Discuss how well it is lived in terms of nurses' attitudes, norms of behavior, use of language, symbols and artifacts, decision making, and sense of belonging. Be specific and provide examples.
3. How does the interviewing process at your health system encourage enculturation of "appropriate" professional practice? How do you know? What could be done differently during interviewing to better facilitate enculturation of the model?
4. Think about your unit. Approximately, how many nurses are at each stage of progression as depicted in Table 9.1. What can you do to facilitate more efficient progression?
5. How does your health system facilitate talent development? Be specific and provide examples. Does it work in terms of enculturation of the PPM? What can be done differently?
6. Suggest three ideas that you could suggest to ensure accountability for the PPM. How could you spread these ideas to coworkers?
7. How could you work together with the nurse leader on your unit to better enculturate the PPM? Provide examples.
8. Name at least two examples of how you live the PPM in your health system.

For Nurse Leaders

1. Who in your organization is responsible for socializing and resocializing nurses? How do they work in tandem to facilitate enculturation? How do you know? Why is this significant?
2. What norms of behavior do you expect nurses in your health system to display in relation to the PPM? Be specific. How do you communicate these expectations, recognize their performance, and facilitate their improvement?
3. Think about three recent nurse hires. Discuss whether they culturally "fit" within the system. How do you know? How does their individual cultural fit limit or enable the delivery of the PPM?
4. Explain how talent acquisition, onboarding, and talent development at your health system ensure enculturation of the PPM. Are any upgrades in these processes needed? What are they? What is your responsibility for contributing to such improvements?

5. What are competency maps? How could you use this talent development approach to enhance enculturation of the PPM? Can you identify someone in the organization that you could work with on this?

6. What novel talent development approaches might you try to facilitate enculturation?

7. Explain how you might raise accountability among direct care nurses for delivering nursing care according to the PPM. What signs would lead you to think that nurses already own the PPM? Why? What can be done to increase ownership of the PPM?

8. Provide an example from your health system's onboarding program that works in terms of enculturation of the PPM. Is it regularly implemented? After reading this chapter, would you change your approach? Why or why not?

9. Discuss the relationship between enculturation of a PPM and nurse engagement. Do you think one influences the other? How could you demonstrate this relationship?

10. List some ways you uphold your ethical responsibility for professional practice environments. What evidence exists for this? What incentives and consequences exist that sustain nursing professional practice? Provide an example of each from your health system.

11. As a nurse leader, how do you live the PPM? What values is it tied to? How could you better facilitate the adoption of the PPM in your health system?

12. How do you work with the human resources department to better enculturate the PPM?

For Nurse Educators

1. How can undergraduate and graduate students best learn about the requirements for socialization and resocialization in a health system?

2. What learning strategies will you use to help students understand the notion of "cultural fit?" What examples will you provide?

3. Develop at least three objectives for a course on health system enculturation targeted at nurse leaders. What evaluation methods will you use?

4. How could you begin to help undergraduate nursing students better understand the interviewing and onboarding processes they will face upon graduation? What learning strategies would you use?

5. How could you work together with other faculty members to help undergraduate students better grasp the concept of accountability for nursing practice? What about graduate students?

6. What specific experiences, exposures, or challenges would you recommend to help students at all levels to better prepare for future career transitions?
7. Do you use competency maps in your curriculum? Why or why not?
8. How might you design a study to examine the contribution of a talent development approach to effective delivery of a PPM? What dependent variable(s) would you include?
9. How could you contribute to the evidence base for PPM enculturation?

LEARNING FROM THE FIELD: HOW OUR PROFESSIONAL PRACTICE MODEL BECAME A MAGNET® EXEMPLAR

In 2014, Texas Health Arlington Memorial Hospital (THAM) received initial Magnet® designation with five exemplars. One exemplar, the enculturation of a new nursing professional practice model (PPM), is the subject of this story and is an accomplishment we are proud to share. Over 1 year earlier, Texas Health Resources (THR) created the PPM with the input and involvement of direct care nurses, nursing educators, and nursing leaders. We wanted our PPM to be meaningful to direct care nurses and illustrate the spirit of nursing in order to advance our profession and improve the health of those we serve. Bedside nurse engagement included a vote by all system nurses on a theorist to be part of the model. Because THR's slogan is "Healing Hands. Caring Hearts," the illustration of the model incorporates hands and hearts. The heart represents system values of respect, integrity, compassion, and excellence. The hands are the nursing actions of teamwork, professional development, shared decision making, and the theoretical foundation of our PPM, the Quality-Caring Model© (Duffy, 2013). Each component creates a meaningful illustration of the nursing care delivered every day by THR nurses (see Figure 7.3 in Chapter 7).

During the implementation phase, educating all nurses about the PPM was deemed necessary and became an important strategy. Solid commitment from our chief nursing officer (CNO) and nursing leadership was a key ingredient in our success. The CNO and/or other nursing leaders facilitated all 80 PPM classes; and because of budgetary/scheduling accommodations, approximately two thirds of nurses were able to attend. Classes were offered at various times during the day, night, and on weekends so that no nurse would miss the chance to be part of the transformation. Instructors provided real-life examples of all of the components of the PPM during interactive lectures in which humor and role-playing permitted nurses to see the PPM behaviors in action. Direct care nurses are often so busy with complicated nursing care tasks that their nursing values and ideals often seem lost: these interactive PPM classes renewed nurses' feelings of pride in their profession and empowerment in their delivery of nursing care.

The last phase of integration was the aspect that impressed Magnet appraisers the most: enculturation. Appraisers noticed that our PPM was everywhere—on mouse pads, templates for agendas and minutes, e-mail signature blocks, and framed PPM images found on all units. Each unit had activities focusing on the hands of the model, where nurses identified examples of teamwork, professional development, shared decision making, and caring. Nurses were able to describe behaviors already practiced that were visible and consistent with the PPM. Duffy's Quality-Caring Model was deeply meaningful to these dedicated nurses who are at high risk for self-care deficit. Nurses identified simple but significant interventions in quality-caring relationships with patients, families, and the health care team.

Even after achieving an exemplar for enculturation of our model, we are continuing the process. Our hospital is leading the way in creating a new system-wide nursing peer evaluation based on components of the model. System leaders are rewriting nursing job descriptions to reflect the PPM. At THAM, all of the components of the THR PPM live in every patient interaction, every family conference, and every nursing intervention carried out by the nurses of THR.

Mary Teague
Debbie Manns
Martha Sleutel

REFERENCES

Advisory Board Company. (2014). *A data driven approach to nurse engagement: Key insights and best practices from the experts.* Retrieved March 4, 2015, from http:// www.advisory.com/~/media/Advisory-com/Research/NEC/Events/ Webconference/2014/Data-Driven-Approach-to-Nurse-Engagement-040914 .pdf

Bauer, T. N. (2010). *Onboarding new employees: Maximizing success.* Alexandria, VA: Society for Human Resource Management Foundation. Retrieved February 23, 2015, from http://www.shrm.org/about/foundation/products/Documents/ Onboarding%20EPG-%20FINAL.pdf

Bauer, T. N. (2013). Onboarding: The power of connection. Retrieved March 3, 2015, from https://drive.google.com/file/d/0Bx-CW4kNTDvYb200Y3V1TWo0d2M/edit

Bradt, G., & Vonnegut, M. (2009). *Onboarding: How to get your new employees to speed up in less than half the time*. Hoboken, NJ: John Wiley & Sons.

Cable, D. M., Gino, F., & Staats, B. R. (2013). Breaking them in or eliciting their best? Reframing socialization around newcomers' authentic self-expression. *Administrative Science Quarterly, 58*(1), 1–36.

Capaldo, G., Landoli, L., & Zollo, G. (2006), A situationalist perspective to competency management, *Human Resource Management, 45*(3), 429–448.

Chao, G. T., O'Leary-Kelly, A. M., Wolf, S., Klein, H. J., & Gardner, P. D. (1994). Organizational socialization: its content and consequences. *Journal of Applied Psychology, 79*(5), 730–743.

Clifford, S. (2006). The new science of hiring. *Inc.com, 28*(8), 90–98.

Dierdorff, E. C., Rubin, R. S., & Morgeson, F. P. (2009). The milieu of managerial work: an integrative framework linking work context to role requirements. *Journal of Applied Psychology, 94*(4), 972–988.

Duffy, J. (2013). *Quality caring in nursing and health systems: Implications for clinical practice, education, and leadership*. New York, NY: Springer Publishing Company.

Gagné, F. (2000). Understanding the complex choreography of talent development. In K. A. Heller, F. J. Mönks, R. J. Sternberg, & R. F. Subotnik, (Eds.), *International handbook of giftedness and talent* (pp. 67–80). Oxford, UK: Elsevier.

Garavan, T. N., Carbery, R., & Rock, A. (2012). Mapping talent development: Definition, scope and architecture. *European Journal of Training and Development, 36*(1), 5–24.

Garazonik, R., Nethersell, G., & Spreier, S. (2006). Navigating through the new leadership landscape. *Leader to Leader, 39*, 30–39.

Hall, A. (2013). "I'm outta here!" Why 2 million Americans quit every month (and 5 steps to turn the epidemic around). *Forbes.com*. Retrieved February 20, 2015, from http://www.forbes.com/sites/alanhall/2013/03/11/im-outta-here-why-2-million-americans-quit-every-month-and-5-steps-to-turn-the-epidemic-around/

Hoebel, E. A. (1949). *Man in the primitive world*. New York, NY: McGraw-Hill.

Huffcutt, A. I., Van Iddekingeb, C. H., & Roth, P. L. (2011). Understanding applicant behavior in employment interviews: A theoretical model of interviewee performance. *Human Resource Management Review, 21*(4), 353–367.

Isrealite, L. (2010). Thinking about talent. In L. Israelite (Ed.), *Talent management strategies for success from six leading companies* (pp. 1–14). Boston, MA: ASTD Press.

Jamka, B. (2011). Values vs. the diversity management business model. *Management and Business Administration, Central Europe, 19*(6), 65–75.

Johns, G. (2006). The essential impact of context on organizational behavior. *Academy of Management Review, 31*(2), 386–408.

Kahn, W. A. (1990). Psychological conditions of personal engagement and disengagement at work. *Academy Management Journal, 33,* 692–724.

Keydo, K. (2014). Work engagement in nursing practice: A relational ethics perspective *Nursing Ethics, 21*(8), 879–889.

Mackintosh, C. (2006). Caring: The socialization of pre-registration student nurses: a longitudinal qualitative descriptive study. *International Journal of Nursing Studies, 43*(8), 953–962.

Michaels, E., Handfield-Jones, H., & Axelrod, B. (2001). *The war for talent.* Boston, MA: Harvard Business Review Press.

Neiterman, E., & Bourgeault, I. L. (2015). Professional integration as a process of professional resocialization: Internationally educated health professionals in Canada. *Social Science in Medicine, 131,* 74–81.

Price, S. L. (2009). Becoming a nurse: A meta-study of early professional socialization and career choice in nursing. *Journal of Advanced Nursing, 65*(1), 11–19.

Schaufeli, W. B., Salanova, M., González-Romá, V., & Bakker, A. B. (2002). The measurement of engagement and burnout: a two sample confirmatory factor analytic approach. *Journal of Happiness Studies, 3*(1), 71–92.

Seligman, M. E. P., Steen, T., Park, N., & Peterson, C. (2005). Positive psychology progress: Empirical validation of interventions. *American Psychologist, 60*(5), 410–421.

Tutlas, C. A. (2011). Enculturation of professional contract nurses: A concept analysis. *Nursing Economic$, 29*(1), 24–31.

Vinje, H. F., & Mittelmark, M. B. (2008). Community nurses who thrive: The critical role of job engagement in the face of adversity. *Journal of Nurses in Staff Development, 24*(5), 195–202.

Workitect. (2012). *Competency develop guide.* Fort Lauderdate, FL: Author.

PART III

From Application to Impact

CHAPTER **10**

Enduring Professional Practice Models: Sustainment

KEY WORDS

Sustainability, organizational memory

OBJECTIVES

By the end of this chapter, readers will be able to:

1. Define the nurse leader's role in the long-term sustainment of a professional practice model (PPM)
2. Evaluate various sustainability frameworks and assessment tools
3. Analyze the term *organizational memory*
4. State at least four leadership strategies used to enhance sustainability of PPMs

THE NATURE OF SUSTAINABILITY

Although a PPM may become internalized such that professional nurses reinterpret the nature of nursing practice according to its components, embed it in daily workflow, and assume accountability for its appropriate delivery, its long-term survival in a health system is not ensured.

In fact, in the face of adjustments (in this case, behavior changes), many individuals are prone to returning to older, more familiar behaviors and, as the initial enthusiasm wanes and competing demands begin to dominate leaders' time, many often fail to recognize their important role in this phase of integration. In fact, without active engagement, continued support, and dedicated attention, sustaining a professional practice model (PPM) over the long term often lapses after implementation is completed. Upholding a PPM over time, however, is necessary to positively impact health outcomes and demonstrate value for a health system. Furthermore, it represents an organization's investment in the PPM and as such, warrants ongoing upkeep.

Sustainability refers to the continual presence of all or most of an innovation's (e.g., PPM) components so that delivery of its intended benefits over an extended period of time can be realized after implementation support has been terminated (Blasinsky, Goldman, & Untzer, 2006; Shediac-Rizkallah & Bone, 1998). The importance of sustaining a PPM so that its usefulness and value can be demonstrated is crucial. Too many health care innovations are left inadequately integrated and, despite major investments of time and resources, their intended results often remain unknown to clinicians, health systems, or worse, to patients and families.

Some studies have illustrated the difficulties of sustaining new programs but few have systematically investigated the concept. However, in one systematic review, partial sustainability was reported to be more common than full sustainability, an increase in the number of recipient-level benefits was reported, and fidelity to the original innovation was incomplete (Stirman et al., 2012). Additionally, the evidence for sustainability was reported to be immature and fragmented, limiting knowledge advancement. In spite of this, understanding the challenges related to sustainability of innovations and testing various strategies for long-term sustainment could never be more necessary. Some authors have provided frameworks concerning sustainability that may help foster research and more effective integration.

SUSTAINABILITY FRAMEWORKS

The public health discipline has provided several frameworks for considering the concept of sustainability. For example, Schell and colleagues (2013) referred to specific factors that influence sustainability, particularly related to chronic disease innovations for community application. Using a comprehensive literature review, input from an expert panel, and the results of concept mapping, a number of selected factors were identified that represent the core domains of capacity for public health program sustainability. They include environmental support, funding stability, partnerships, organizational capacity, program evaluation, program adaptation, communications, and strategic planning. The authors suggest that these factors may be related to a program's ability to sustain its activities and benefits over time and may be useful for decision makers, program managers, program evaluators, and implementation researchers.

Another contribution from the public health literature is the sustainability planning model (Johnson, Hays, Hayden, & Daley, 2004), also known as intervention theory. This model is a comprehensive, prescriptive, capacity-building approach that denotes a group of factors (e.g., type of structure and formal linkages, presence of champions for an innovation, effective leadership, resources, administrative policies and procedures, and expertise), innovation attributes (e.g., alignment with needs, positive relationships among key implementers, successful implementation and effectiveness in the target system, and ownership by system stakeholders), and actions that need to be addressed to explain sustainability readiness and ultimately sustainability outcomes (e.g., integration of an innovation into normal operations at the organizational, community, state, or federal levels and key stakeholders' benefits received as a result of the innovation). The relationship between innovation integration into a system and stakeholder benefits is considered reciprocal in this framework, with each outcome influencing the other.

From a broader organizational view, Yin's routinization framework (1979, 1981) was developed after examining how technical innovations became standard practice. Yin refers to sustainability as the institutionalization or routinization of programs into ongoing organizational core services. Yin suggested that full routinization depends on processes or cycles and distinguishes among three degrees of routinization: marginal, moderate, and high, reflecting the number of cycles that had been encountered. Some examples of routinization cycles (Yin, 1979, 1981) are as follows:

- The new program survives annual budget cycles.
- Program activities become part of job descriptions/hiring practices.
- The program survives turnover of personnel/leadership.
- Key program staff members are promoted within the agency.
- Supply and maintenance are provided by the agency.
- It is spread throughout the system (or niche saturation).
- Many training cycles are observed.
- Competencies become part of professional standards.
- The use of the program is recognized in manuals, procedures, meeting minutes, and regulations.
- The innovation is recognized as permanent within the agency.

In this way, the new program becomes unidentifiable as it is blended into the institutional infrastructure.

In another framework, Racine (2006) names three sets of factors—innovation legitimacies, contextual conditions (organizationally and locally), and functional attributes such as technical competence and communication influencing sustainment of innovations. The usefulness, relevance, acceptability, and, most important, the value of an innovation, which consistently delivers on these factors, demonstrate an innovation's legitimacy. The local and organizational fit with the innovation and employee functional attributes also play important roles in sustained effectiveness of innovations.

Although these frameworks help to better understand the complex nature of sustaining new programs, they have several limitations. For example, there is little discussion of costs or contexts, and they refer to sustainment in a linear fashion (which is often not the case in the complex world of health care).

The challenge of implementing multicomponent innovations, such as a PPM in complex, dynamic health systems, presumes that a well-developed implementation plan followed by evaluation and ongoing leadership support will ensure successful and lasting integration. Yet, the ever changing health care context often limits such sustainability. The Dynamic Sustainability Framework (DSF), however, acknowledges that change is constant and sustainability of an innovation over time requires ongoing development and refinement that is never complete (Chambers, Glasgow, & Stange, 2013).

In this way of imagining sustainability, the PPM, already enculturated within a health system, benefits from continued improvement that allows potential enhancements to be made and shared, offering better information on which to make decisions to cease old ways of delivering care. The intention is to recognize and support rapid learning, real-time problem solving, and generation of knowledge, through a shared process of continual experimentation and analysis, not just routine application of a static PPM.

The DSF is intended to suggest a new longer term paradigm with ongoing improvement of the PPM (even pooling of data from multiple sites), allowing continuous exposure of the innovation to new populations and new contexts. Indeed, the DSF posits that ongoing improvement is the ultimate aim, with optimization of the fit between the model and the dynamic delivery context essential to achieving sustainment. Although this framework is more dynamic, the question of sustainability of a PPM in health systems may also be understood through more practical behaviors observed in most organizations.

Organizational Memory

As suggested by several sustainability frameworks, shared knowledge, actions, or practices (organizational routines) play a key role in innovation continuance. One of those shared traditions, namely, organizational memory, is defined as shared interpretations of past experiences that are brought to bear on present activities (Stein, 1995). Furthermore, Walsh and Ungson (1991) asserted that organizational memory is not stored centrally but is distributed across different retention facilities. It refers to the collective ability to acquire, store, and retrieve knowledge and information. This persistence of organizational traits over time suggests that retention and transmission of information (or knowledge) from past generations to future members of a system is intact. This is important for organizations because it represents the "personality" of the system (Weick, 1979) and preserves its autonomy (Deutsch, 1966). In essence, the memories maintained by an organization plot a map of the past that contains information crucial to organizational effectiveness (Stein, 1995).

In terms of significant experiences, organizations "remember" lessons from the past in a variety of ways. An organization's memory resides in the minds of individual employees, in their many relationships with each other, in repositories, such as computer databases and file cabinets, and can also be embedded in work processes that have evolved over time. For example, in nursing, the routine of admitting a new patient into a hospital may be "remembered" as a unique series of tasks that involves specific individuals and reflects lessons learned about admission over time. This collective knowledge is then transmitted to each new generation of nurses in such a way that allows for little deviation from those past experiences.

Thus, organizational memory is neither good nor bad, but it sets the tone for a system, affecting employee attitudes and behaviors, and ultimately its success.

Stein (1995) proposed that organizational memory is associated with organizational effectiveness, and the processes of acquisition, retention, maintenance, and retrieval are necessary for organizational memory to operate.

Because they vary from one system to the next, higher or lower levels of organizational memory are created. For example, memories are acquired through learning over time, recorded events, and are retained within individuals or groups of people who work together for a long time, and through certain rituals or ceremonies. They are maintained through specific norms and artifacts, including logos, symbols, or designs, and are retrievable through individuals, written documents, and observations of specific routines. Such memories can enhance or thwart long-term sustainability of innovations.

Organizational memory as it relates to a PPM refers to what organizations learn, reminisce about, and recollect as they experience it. If organizational memory about professional practice is congruent with organizational values and mission, this can lead to long-lasting performance that may advantage the system over its competitors. Contrarily, if it evokes negative memories, it can threaten the practice, leading to fragmentation or inappropriate behaviors, and its chances for extended survival are less likely because employees' "remembered" routines may undermine the new innovation, damaging the system's ability to deliver long term. Thus, the long-term sustainability of a PPM may be dependent on organizational memories about what nursing means in the model and how it was applied. Nevertheless, because organizational memory resides in individuals and groups of individuals, it can easily fall apart.

For example, as systems lose employees, restructure, realign purposes, or add innovations to meet new demands, the shared knowledge and routines accumulated over time begin to collapse. For leaders, organizational memory is a system characteristic that must be respected and, in the case of a PPM, leveraged for future decision making. For instance, identifying ahead of time which experiences vis-à-vis the PPM hold important lessons for future nurses helps direct efforts to preserve such knowledge. For example, important learning events that are critical, one-of-a-kind opportunities, such as inaugural presentations, inspirational messages, or significant consulting engagements during which unique approaches were discussed, should be preserved through archived means. Assigning appropriate champions and role models who will facilitate integration in a relationship-friendly manner gradually helps nurses develop new skills and embeds these new behaviors into routine practices. Noticing, naming, and documenting relevant practices in which the PPM is entrenched ensure that the lessons of experience influence how nursing work is remembered for future generations. The main leadership challenge consists of establishing what needs to be preserved and how that preservation will drive nursing work in the future, ultimately creating long-lasting value for the health system. In doing so, the benefits of good organizational memory may be realized:

- It can help leaders and leaders of the future uphold intentional direction over time.
- It can facilitate access to the choice, design, implementation, and evaluation of the model as it was first encountered, providing meaning to the work of individual nurses.
- It can strengthen the identity of the health system.
- It can enable health systems to avoid past mistakes.
- It can enable use of best practices.
- It can provide newcomers with access to the expertise of those who preceded them.

> In essence, nurse leaders can continue to influence future nurse work by deliberately developing good organizational memories and using those pockets of knowledge to guide organizational activities and decision making over time.

A health system's *capacity* for sustainment, however, might be assessed through specific tracking and sustainability measures.

MEASURING SUSTAINABILITY

Although individual health systems and researchers create unique approaches for evaluating sustainability of new programs, services, and innovations, many are not routinely applied, validity and reliability are often not reported, and many are inaccurately administered. Because some theoretical work has already been conducted on sustainability (see sustainability frameworks, described previously), acceptable precision is available to guide the evaluation of sustainability, albeit it tends to be very specific to a population. For example, the Program Sustainability Assessment Tool (PSAT; Luke, Calhoun, Robichaux, Elliott, & Moreland-Russell, 2014) derived from the program sustainability framework (Schell, 2013) has been reported ($N = 592$). This instrument contains 40 items, has eight domains, with five items per domain. Confirmatory factor analysis shows good fit of the data and the subscales have excellent internal consistency, ranging from .79 to .92 with the overall Cronbach's α = .88. Although seemingly easy to use, validation is ongoing.

Similarly, Goodman, McLeroy, Steckler, and Hoyle (1993) used Yin's (1979) routinization framework to develop the Level of Institutionalization Scales (LoIn) of health-promotion programs. The LoIn instrument is a beginning effort to measure the extent of program integration in organizations. A questionnaire designed to test this construct was mailed to 453 administrators in 141 organizations that operate health-promotion programs in North Carolina. Based on a 71% response rate, a confirmatory factor analysis supported an eight-factor structure: four factors concerned how routinized the program was in each subsystem and four factors concerned the degree of program saturation within each subsystem. Correlations of the eight factors with the number of years the programs had been in operation, and managers' perceptions of program permanency, indicated that the four routinization factors were more highly correlated with program longevity than the four niche saturation factors, and the niche saturation factors were more highly correlated with managers' perceptions of program permanence than the routinization factors. The instrument, which has 15 items, is a beginning effort to operationalize the degree of routinization and warrants further research and validation in other contexts.

Mancini and Marek (2004) developed a 29-item Program Sustainability Index (PSI) to assess six factors related to the sustainability of community-based programs. They are leadership competence, effective collaboration, demonstrating program results, strategic funding, staff involvement and integration, and program responsivity. Internal consistency among the factors was acceptable: leadership competence ($\alpha = .81$, 5 items), effective collaboration ($\alpha = .88$, 10 items), staff involvement and integration ($\alpha = .76$, 4 items), demonstrating program results ($\alpha = .85$, 4 items), strategic funding ($\alpha = .76$, 3 items), and program responsivity ($\alpha = .67$, 3 items). The researchers used a fairly homogeneous group ($N = 242$) to test the PIS with 242 respondents yielding a promising measure. However, further research is needed with a larger and more diversified population to refine the instrument.

According to Stirman et al. (2012), qualitative and mixed methodologies that assess potential influences across multiple levels of sustainability will continue to be necessary to better understand the relationships between sustainability drivers, and facilitate the development of interventions to promote sustainability. In their review, they suggested that certain qualitative studies yielded a wider variety of findings and highlighted processes and constructs that warrant further study. However, most did not provide interview guides, limiting interpretability and replicability. Thus, although several sustainability measures exist, the development and improvement of the measures will promote better understanding and more effective evaluation.

ENHANCING SUSTAINABILITY

Sustainability cannot be easily addressed after it is finished; rather, it is important to make it a priority from the very beginning of PPM integration.

> Although sustainability may seem to be the natural consequence of successful enculturation, often the gains realized and ongoing evolution (improvement) required are not extended to other contexts or continued over time. Nurse leaders and system administrators can become quite frustrated when they observe that their great efforts to achieve system integration cannot be retained.

Yet, it is imperative to anchor or to have "stickability" to sustain major practice changes and to realize their resultant contribution to system value, such that they become irreversible (Kotter, 1995). Kotter warns that sustainability of innovation is really about culture change and may take 5 to 10 years of enforcing a continued clear vision, and maintenance of the sense of urgency that originally inspired the PPM, new behaviors rooted in norms and values, a clearly understood link between behaviors and performance, and new leaders who continue to champion the changes introduced by their predecessors. Selected recommendations for sustainability of innovation from Scheirer's (2005) review of empirical studies include:

- Choose programs and interventions that relate strongly to a system's mission and culture, so that support from upper management will be likely, and tasks needed to integrate the program will fit within the workloads of available staff members.
- Engage in thoughtful modifications of innovation components to fit the organizational context, without destroying the core components contributing to the effectiveness of the original design.
- Identify and support a program champion to take a leadership role in both initial program development and sustainability planning.
- Emphasize the innovation's benefits for various groups of stakeholders, including staff members and clients, as well as its fit with the major objectives of potential external funders.
- Consider the possible advantages of "routinizing" the program into core operations of the existing system rather than applying it as a "stand-alone" program.
- Use Yin's (1979, 1981) list of factors contributing to routinization as a checklist of organizational aspects to work on.

Other strategies gathered from personal experiences that can facilitate sustainability of PPMs include:

- Celebrate continued successes (e.g., an outcome that has persistently demonstrated a high degree of quality).
- Reflect periodically on the team's progress (e.g., where we were and how far we have come).
- Set "stretch" goals and try to improve even more.
- Find ways to renew the passion for the PPM (e.g., an annual renewal activity).
- Remain consistent over time, never bending from the initial inspiration that drove the model's inception.
- Appropriately manage persistent conceptions of nursing practice.
- Build organizational memory of the PPM.
- Prepare a succession plan so that new leaders and champions are equipped to promote the model's endurance.

In summary, sustainability is a complex process that occurs over time and is subject to unique influences such as leadership, context, employee competence, local political and cultural norms, as well as system-level structures and procedures. Despite several conceptual frameworks and assessment tools, its definition remains unclear and no generalized prescription for sustainability has emerged. In a recent concept analysis, Fleiszer, Semenic, Ritchie, Richer, and Denis (2015) proposed that three characteristics, namely, benefits, routinization or institutionalization, and development comprised the concept. They also suggested influencing factors that are related to innovation, context, leadership, and process affect sustainability, and urged more investigation. Nevertheless, various leadership strategies have been identified and experienced that may advance sustainability of new practices. Much more needs to be done to better understand sustainability of innovations and to prepare leaders for their important role in the process.

SUMMARY

The nature of sustainability was described, including definitions, challenges, and its importance in demonstrating the value of PPMs. Several sustainability frameworks were presented that analyzed influencing factors, capacity-building approaches, institutionalization, and continued improvement as ways of conceptualizing the process. Organizational memory as a set of shared traditions that systems develop over time was reviewed and linked to sustainability. Leaders' roles in preserving organizational memory related to PPMs and its many benefits were espoused. Measuring sustainability was evaluated in terms of psychometric properties and limitations for use. Finally, leadership strategies were offered related to enhancing sustainability and continued research was recommended.

REFLECTIVE APPLICATIONS

For Students

1. Differentiate among the terms *sustainability* and *organizational memory*.
2. Why is sustainability of a PPM so important? How might it affect your long-term performance?
3. Explain how the public health discipline has contributed to our understanding of sustainability.
4. Analyze Schell's sustainability-influencing factors. Provide a positive and negative example of each factor that could affect sustainability of a PPM.
5. Reflect on the measurement tools presented in this chapter. What are your thoughts about using them for assessing sustainability of a PPM? Please explain.
6. What evidence would you expect to see if a PPM was sustained within a health system? Why?
7. Discuss how you can best prepare for sustainment of innovations in your future career.
8. Provide two examples of what you would look for in a leader regarding sustaining innovations. How would you assess these qualities? How could you work together with the nurse leader to ensure sustainability of a PPM?

For Clinical Nurses

1. Discuss why sustainability of innovation is important. Provide an example from your own practice.
2. Analyze the PPM in your health system. Discuss how long it has continued and what evidence exists for its long-term survival. Be specific and provide examples.
3. How does the leadership team in your health system ensure sustainability of new programs? How do you know? Based on the knowledge you acquired from reading this chapter, what could be done differently to better facilitate sustainability?
4. Think about your unit. What organizational memories exist regarding appropriate nursing practice? Are they enhancing or limiting in terms of current professional standards? How do they inform present practice? What can you do to facilitate positive organizational memory?

5. What does the promotion of key PPM supporters demonstrate about sustainability? Why?

6. Suggest three ideas that you could implement to promote sustainability for the PPM at your institution. How could you get coworkers or leaders involved?

7. Name at least two examples of how you sustain the PPM in your health system.

For Nurse Leaders

1. Who in your organization is responsible for sustaining the PPM? Why is such sustainment important?

2. What norms of behavior or other evidence would you expect to observe in your health system if the PPM was continued 10 years from now? Be specific.

3. Discus the statement "sustained practice using the health system's PPM represents the organization's investment." What does this mean to you? How does nursing leadership meet its responsibility regarding the organization's investment in the PPM?

4. Explain how a nurse leader can promote sustainability of a PPM a priori. What would he or she have to do?

5. Analyze the Yin (1979) framework of routinization. How could you use it to enhance sustainability? What are its limitations? Can you identify someone in the organization whom you could work with on this?

6. Explain how surviving a budget cycle (or two) contributes to sustainability of a PPM.

7. Describe why organizational memory is important to PPM sustainability. What organizational memory exists in your health system that could enhance or hinder PPM sustainability? Be specific and provide examples of each. What is your role regarding organizational memory?

8. How does turnover affect organizational memory? What about retention? Why?

9. What signs would lead you to think that sustainability of the PPM will occur? Why? What can be done to improve sustainability of the PPM?

10. Discuss the PSAT and the LoIn measures of sustainability. On which framework were they built? How could you use these to assess sustainability of the PPM in your health system? Or could you? Choose the one you most prefer. Why? How often would you use it? What would you do with the results? Why?

11. Discuss Kotter's (1995) "stickability" concept. Using the leader strategies listed in this chapter, suggest at least three specific activities you could use to enhance stickability of the PPM.

For Nurse Educators

1. How could you best help undergraduate students learn about the sustainability of health care innovations? Is this important for them to understand? What about graduate students?
2. What evidence would you suggest could be used to demonstrate sustainability? How might that apply to your current curriculum?
3. Develop at least three learning objectives for a lecture on the DSF. What evaluation methods will you use to ensure its comprehension and application?
4. Develop a brief interview guide to assess sustainability of a PPM. How would you use it? What learning strategies would you use to assist nurse leaders in its administration?
5. What organizational memory exists in your program? How does it enhance or limit current faculty behavior? Be specific, providing examples of each. How could you help create new organizational memory related to innovations in curriculum?
6. What specific experiences, exposures, or challenges would you recommend to help nurse leaders better prepare for their roles related to sustainability of health care innovations?
7. Develop a research question that would examine the concept of sustainability. Do you see yourself pursuing this line of study? Why or why not?
8. How could the measurement tools described in this chapter be applied in your program? Should they?

LEARNING FROM THE FIELD: PROFESSIONAL PRACTICE MODEL SUSTAINABILITY

Sustainability Starts With Development

Similar to preparing for patient discharge from the point of admission, sustainability of a professional practice model (PPM) starts with development. However, developing the PPM can be challenging. When conducted in a thoughtful manner, however, capturing the values of the nurses who work within an organization in an authentic manner, the end result is a practice model that is more sustainable than those composed in boardrooms with catch phrases that resonate only in the executive "C" suite. A model that speaks to the true intentions of clinical nurses is easier to remember and will naturally flow into everyday practice. To do this, the responsibility for creating, maintaining, and evaluating professional nursing practice should reside with clinical nurses with support from leadership.

Remembering nursing values may be assisted through the use of a mnemonic positioned strategically around the model image. For instance, one coastal organization adopted the image of a starfish because starfish represent autonomous practice while working toward common goals, which clinical nurses equated to their beliefs about shared governance. One of the clinical nurses on the practice council challenged the team to select shared key values from the organization's values, mission, vision, the Quality-Caring Model© (Duffy, 2009, 2013), and the nursing strategic plan that would spell *starfish*. These words would become the key elements within the practice model. The council put forward suggestions that were amended through an iterative voting structure and then adopted by the organization. Although eight values (the number of letters in the word *starfish*) are a lot to remember, using the mnemonic supports memory.

Delegation Improves Dissemination

After deciding on the key values, the image, and then writing the accompanying philosophy statements, the hard work is to strategically analyze what needs to change in order to make the model come alive. The practice model needs to be transformed from inanimate words on a page to the living, breathing practice of every nurse in the organization. The practice council, which may be primarily responsible for developing, reviewing, and evaluating the practice model, needs to delegate tasks to other groups and councils. Delegating serves two purposes. First, many hands make light work. More important, every group that engages in an activity to launch and sustain the model becomes intimately aware of the details of how it affects clinical practice and nursing leadership.

Update Key Documents and Programs

The first step is to make a list of key practice guidelines, and ask their authors to review them in the context of the practice model and make the associated changes. Setting a deadline for proposed changes to be returned to the practice council enhances efficiency. Key organizational programs, such as new graduate residency and orientation, need to be evaluated and updated so that all new employees are routinely indoctrinated into the values of the organization. These changes heavily affect the department of education, and their practice council representative should provide a departmental briefing on these responsibilities and prepare a timeline for completion of the work, gently reminding colleagues when work is due.

Posting signage of the practice model image is common, yet less likely to produce lasting results. The image may be reproduced as screen savers, mouse pads, on pens with the organization's logo, and on meeting-minute agendas. Template slide sets for presentations may also insert the model on the title slide for increased visibility. Making these graphic changes and preparing the artwork to operationalize the plan requires collaboration with the marketing department. These imaging strategies make the practice model accessible where all staff has access to it without searching, but are not quite as powerful as learning through living examples of those who practice the model.

Following internal imaging, the outward-facing profile of nursing on the Internet should be evaluated for potential changes to consciously attract nurses who align themselves with the key values within the model. This usually requires collaboration with the marketing department and/or image council.

Criteria for clinical ladder enhancement should be reviewed to identify how to promote projects and activities aligned to the model. This portion of the project may be delegated to the professional development council.

There is likely an existing nursing strategic plan that should be evaluated by its authors to ensure that the objectives and goals within the plan are aligned to the model. It is possible that a new or updated PPM highlights a value that was not focused on in the past. Ensure that the updated value in the model is reflected with an activity or goal within the strategic plan.

The PPM should be transparent enough that the people served know about nursing's key values and intentions of practice. This can be accomplished in the form of standardized welcome information, including information about the PPM and also amending the initial assessment to include key phrases addressing the practice model. For instance, if the Quality-Caring Model (Duffy, 2009, 2013) is adopted as a theoretical framework, the patient admission assessment can be prompted to encourage a discussion that includes a sentence containing key elements from the model such as, "It is our goal that you feel cared for during every experience you have. No matter how busy we look, we are here to care for you. You can trust us, we are skilled at what we do, and we care."

Nurse researchers can be encouraged to use the underlying PPM nursing framework as a theoretical framework for related studies. If research or evidence-based practice (EBP) conferences are held to promote changes in practice, the abstract application forms can be modified to have prospective presenters explain how the project is aligned to the PPM. The research and/or EBP council may embrace this activity.

Leadership Support Is Necessary to Fund a Launch

According to Bloom's taxonomy (2005), learning occurs best with application and synthesis of key concepts in an interactive multimodal educational program. An official launch is necessary following model design or revision. Nurses benefit from live discussions about the model and what it means to their own practice instead of a read-and-sign in-service or online training module. A launch program should be designed to engage the audience with actual examples of the PPM in action. A blank worksheet can accompany the program on which learners write in "What the Model Means to Me" in various structured learning activities.

Exploratory questions such as these may help:

- Why did we make the change to this PPM?
- How will the PPM make us better nurses?
- How will this PPM move us from good to great?
- What key values are showcased on the PPM?

One at a time, have people stand up if they have engaged in activities that express the value. For instance, if the value is professional development, ask those who are enrolled in a formal educational program to stand up. Then ask anyone who has taught a class to stand up. Then ask those who have been to a program to advance their knowledge to stand up. By the end of the values list, it will be clear which values are most commonly expressed and which are in need of development. Point this out to the audience.

This interactive PPM value assessment illuminates areas of opportunities and validates why the changes, if acted on, will improve the work environment. For instance, one organization adopted the Quality-Caring Model (Duffy, 2009, 2013) because of the emphasis on building caring relationships with each other, starting with caring for self. When groups are asked to "Tell us about a time when you felt cared for at work," there was a pause, reflection, and sometimes a struggle to come up with a recent example. The conversation was then naturally moved to "How can we promote caring behaviors in the workplace toward each other?" Unit leaders were encouraged to focus on teambuilding, team support, and projects to enhance self-care in the workplace. Because the other values were so deeply embedded already and this one was valued highly but less prominent, it became the focus of the first year following the practice model revision.

Reward Those Who Live the Model

Most organizations have a "nurse of the year" program and some have monthly nurse rewards. The criteria for issuing the award can be modified to include the values selected for representation on the practice model image. The exemplars of award winning and nominated clinical nurses can be used for teaching and reflection to promote the behaviors and practices espoused in the model through living examples. When the reflections are presented, if coupled with the picture of a nurse, the result becomes an artistic form of knowing that is more meaningful than the image alone (Carper, 1978). Artistic expressions of the model can also be solicited for display at conferences. Photos of these pieces of art can be used to make card sets to be used for thank-you notes and other forms of positive communication.

Encourage Innovation

So far, predictable forms of embedding the values that drive the practice model into the framework of the organization have been explored. However, if given the challenge, creative clinical nurses and leaders may come up with their own novel or innovative approaches. For instance, after being offered the challenge, the clinical nurse specialist who oversees the emergency response system decided to embed the model within basic and advanced life-support programs. This would naturally refresh model values for every staff member every 2 years. During this program she led the group through a discussion concerning how the caring factors (Duffy, 2009, 2013) are addressed in resuscitation events. Some discussion points could include:

- Affiliation needs: Family presence at resuscitation
- Human respect: Respecting choices about resuscitation that might not be our own
- Attentive reassurance: Debriefing to assure future possibilities and bolster feelings

- Encouraging manner: Emotional support to family during resuscitation and debriefings to provide encouragement to each other
- Basic human needs: Tending to the basic human need to feel safe, not blamed, for the event; acknowledging the need for an emotional break (time out) before going on to the next patient
- Healing environment: Maintaining a professional demeanor during the crisis and with the family; offering debriefing for family and staff; removing evidence of blood/struggle at the earliest opportunity; covering the patient when possible; professional comportment during death; discussion of the patient's contributions following death
- Appreciation of unique meanings: Debriefing to understand why this patient responded the way that he or she did and how that behavior might vary from others
- Mutual problem solving: Team decision making during resuscitation; team debriefing following the resuscitation to identify opportunities for improvement in the future, need for resources, equipment, or training
- Caring relationships: Building the team through team training and team debriefings
- Feeling cared for: Knowing that feeling cared for helps us to take action to engage in self-care activities, "What does it take to feel 'cared for' and supported as an employee after a resuscitation event?" Lead the group in a discussion about the importance of debriefs

CONCLUSIONS

The sustainability of a PPM is dependent on disseminating responsibility widely, and building key nursing values into the fabric of important documents and programs within the organization. A planned launch will help support the penetration of the model into practice. Celebrating those who routinely practice the espoused values encourages others to do the same.

Key Points

- Sustainability starts with development.
- Leadership support is needed to financially support a launch.
- Delegation improves dissemination and integration.
- Evaluate all key programs and documents for needed changes.
- Reward those who live the model.
- Challenge nurses to design innovative strategies for sustaining the model.

Judy E. Davidson

REFERENCES

Blasinsky, M., Goldman, H. H., & Untzer, J. (2006). Project IMPACT: A report on barriers and facilitators to sustainability. *Administration and Policy in Mental Health and Mental Health Services Research, 33*(6), 718–729.

Bloom, B. S. (2005). Effects of continuing medical education on improving physician clinical care and patient health: A review of systematic reviews. *International Journal of Technology Assessment in Health Care, 21*(3), 380–385.

Carper, B. (1978). Fundamental patterns of knowing in nursing. *Advances in Nursing Science 1*(1), 13–23.

Chambers, D. A., Glasgow, R. E., & Stange, K. C. (2013). The dynamic sustainability framework: Addressing the paradox of sustainment amid ongoing change. *Implementation Science, 8*, 117. doi:10.1186/1748-5908-8-117

Deutsch, K. W. (1966). *The nerves of government* (pp. 128–129). New York, NY: Free Press.

Duffy, J. R. (2009). *Quality caring in nursing: Applying theory to clinical practice, education, and leadership.* New York, NY: Springer Publishing Company.

Duffy, J. R. (2013). *Quality caring in nursing and health systems: Implications for clinical practice, education, and leadership.* New York, NY: Springer Publishing Company.

Fleiszer, A. R., Semenic, S. E., Ritchie, J. A., Richer, M., & Denis, J. L. (2015). The sustainability of health care innovations: A concept analysis. *Journal of Advanced Nursing, 71*, 1484–1498. doi:10.1111/jan.12633

Goodman, R. M., McLeroy, K. R., Steckler, A. B., & Hoyle, R. H. (1993). Development of level of institutionalization scales for health promotion programs. *Health Education Quarterly, 20*(2), 161–179.

Johnson, K., Hays, B., Hayden, C., & Daley, C. (2004). Building capacity and sustainable prevention innovations: A sustainability planning model. *Evaluation and Program Planning, 27*(2), 135–149.

Kotter, J. P. (1995). Leading change: Why transformation efforts fail. *Harvard Business Review, 73*(2), 59–67.

Luke, D. A., Calhoun, A., Robichaux, C. B., Elliott, M. B., & Moreland-Russell, S. (2014). The program sustainability assessment tool: A new instrument for public health programs. *Prevention in Chronic Disease, 11*, 130184. Retrieved March 23, 2015, from http://dx.doi.org/10.5888/pcd11.130184

Mancini, J. A., & Marek, L. I. (2004). Sustaining community-based programs for families: Conceptualization and measurement. *Family Relationships, 53*(4), 339–347.

Racine, D. P. (2006). Reliable effectiveness: A theory on sustaining and replicating worthwhile innovations. *Administration and Policy in Mental Health and Mental Health Services Research, 33*(3), 356–387.

Shediac-Rizkallah, M. C., & Bone, L. R. (1998). Planning for the sustainability of community-based health programs: Conceptual frameworks and future directions for research, practice and policy. *Health Education Research, 13*(1), 87–108.

Scheirer, M. A. (2005). Is sustainability possible? A review and commentary on empirical studies of program sustainability. *American Journal of Evaluation*, 26(3), 320–347.

Schell, S. F., Luke, D. A., Schooley, M. W., Elliott, M. B., Herbers, S. H., Mueller, N. B., & Bunger, A. C. (2013). Public health program capacity for sustainability: A new framework. *Implementation Science*, 8, 15. doi:10.1186/1748-5908-8-15

Stein, E. W., (1995). Organizational memory: Review of concepts and recommendations for management. *International Journal of Information Management*, 15(1), 17–32.

Stirman, S. W., Kimberly, J., Cook, N., Calloway, A., Castor, F., & Charns, M. (2012). The sustainability of new programs and innovations: A review of the empirical literature and recommendations for future research. *Implementation Science*, 7, 17. doi:10.1186/1748-5908-7-17

Walsh, J. P., & Ungson, G. R. (1991). Organizational memory. *Academy of Management Review*, 16(1), 57–91.

Weick, K. E. (1979). *The social psychology of organizing* (2nd ed.). Reading, MA: Addison-Wesley.

Yin, R. K. (1979). *Changing urban bureaucracies: How new practices become routinized.* Lexington, MA: Lexington Books.

Yin, R. K. (1981). Life histories of innovations: How new practices become routinized. *Public Administration Review, 41,* 21–28.

CHAPTER 11

Spreading Lessons Learned and Best Practices: Dissemination

KEY WORDS

Spread, lessons learned, best practices, dissemination, scaling up, distribution

OBJECTIVES

By the end of this chapter, readers will be able to:

1. Differentiate between lessons learned and best practices
2. Describe the importance and value of dissemination as it relates to professional practice models (PPMs)
3. Evaluate dissemination frameworks
4. Explain how the term *scaling up* can be applied to lessons learned and best practices
5. List at least three strategies for distributing lessons learned and best practices
6. Describe the role of leadership in dissemination

LESSONS LEARNED AND BEST PRACTICES

The ultimate goal of professional practice model integration is to change practice in health systems such that health outcomes are enhanced for patients and families and the disciplinary values and contributions of nursing are upheld and advanced.

Usually, such integration occurs in a single clinical site in a particular geographic location. Yet, health systems and their employees often learn important lessons through their experiences of implementing and evaluating projects (or innovations) and/or identify best practices as a result of integration processes, but many of these useful implications fade or perish when not promptly shared with others who might benefit.

Lessons learned include both positive and negative understandings gained from the experiences of integrating a professional practice model (PPM) or other large-scale innovations. For example, using a particular evaluation tool might be found to be better (or worse) than another and, if shared with others, could potentially influence decision making. Or a certain educational strategy might be assessed as more efficient at achieving important project outcomes, saving others valuable time. However, noticing and understanding the value of such lessons requires some reflection on the experiences, documentation of the learning points (positive or negative), analysis of the source or basis of the lesson, and recommendations for incorporating the "lesson" in future contexts. Formal lessons learned are typically drawn at the conclusion of projects; however, they can be developed at any time during the integration phases.

> These "lessons" learned from experiences in one health system can advantage others by providing valuable insights, useful and applied processes, information about evaluation methods, and enabling strategies for adaptation and enculturation.

Best practices, on the other hand, have become known in health care from the business world, and include "methods or techniques that have consistently shown results superior to those achieved with other means, and that are used as benchmarks" ("Best practices," 2015). In health care, the World Health Organization (WHO) defined *best practice* as "knowledge about what works in specific situations and contexts, without using inordinate resources to achieve the desired results, and which can be used to develop and implement solutions adapted to similar health problems in other situations and contexts" (WHO, 2008, p. 2). In this definition, "what works" signifies that results of specific processes or strategies are known and can be documented—in other words, adequate evaluation has been conducted. Such "tested" information enables additional health systems to learn how "best" to implement specific strategies, thus preventing the "reinventing the wheel" syndrome or inadvertently duplicating others' mistakes, fostering better effectiveness and efficiency of project outcomes. Although not research per se, effective PPM integration uses implementation and evaluation approaches that require specialized strategies and assessments that consume health system resources; thus, sharing them with others may expedite efficiencies.

> Nurses and nurse leaders who generate lessons learned and best practices from professional practice model integration and who *promptly share* them with others (even if they are negative), promote more widespread application and evaluation in a variety of new settings and populations.

> Health systems that *apply* lessons learned and best practices to professional practice model integration at their sites may be poised to deliver more effective implementation strategies, evaluation techniques, and achieve intended successes, such as improved patient quality outcomes, while ensuring efficiencies of the integration process itself.

However, the dissemination of such information is not typically included as an important component of health systems' PPM integration plans.

DISSEMINATION EXPLAINED

The process of spreading lessons learned and best practices is complex, protracted, and frequently left undone, limiting additional health systems and stakeholders from learning about advantages they could potentially experiment with and reducing opportunities for some health systems to showcase their successes. For example, generating and then rapidly dispersing lessons learned and best practices resulting from PPM integration that could benefit others can be hampered by time requirements and/or lack of experience with publication and presentation, the time from manuscript acceptance to publication, the characteristics of the best practices themselves, and variation in the local contexts of other health systems (e.g., the willingness or ability of others to try the new ideas, or the characteristics of the culture and infrastructure [including resources] of a health system to embrace new ideas). Although reporting about research findings, Colquhoun Aplin, Geary, Goodman, and Hatcher (2012) suggested that the diversity and inconsistency of dissemination terminology and frameworks are an additional barrier to applying findings. Thus, it can sometimes take years and many strained attempts to effectively integrate and sustain PPMs, potentially disadvantaging those patients, families, and health professionals served by additional health systems.

Understanding how to rapidly and effectively spread lessons learned and/or best practices from professional practice model integration in and across complex health systems is vital to more rapidly and pervasively improve patient outcomes and advance professional nursing over a wider range of health systems and geographic settings.

To improve dissemination of best practices, it is essential to understand the term, consider various perspectives and methods used to attain success in broadcasting superior ways of working. *Dissemination* refers to "the targeted distribution of information and practice change materials to a specific public health or clinical practice audience" (Glasgow et al., 2012, p. 1275), representing an active process (Greenhalgh, Robert, MacFarlane, Bate, & Kyriakidou, 2004). More recently, the Patient-Centered Outcomes Research Institute (PCORI) defined *dissemination* as: "the intentional, active process of identifying target audiences and tailoring communication strategies to increase awareness and understanding of evidence, and to motivate its use in policy, practice, and individual choices" (Esposito, Heeringa, Bradley, Croake, & Kimmey, 2015, p. 3). The ultimate purpose of dissemination is to increase impact (McNichol & Grimshaw, 2014), implying that the new findings, lessons learned, or best practices, are *applied or used* and evaluated in additional sites or with different individuals.

In the case of nursing PPMs, the clinical practice audience includes similar clinical sites beyond the original site (e.g., extension to a health system or close regional sites), clinical sites within a different context (e.g., best practices learned in acute care and applied to community-based sites [home care, extended care, primary care]), and the discipline as a whole (e.g., rapid dissemination nationally and internationally). How do lessons learned and best practices from one health system best reach others beyond the original site, in alternative contexts, or effectively and efficiently inform the discipline?

The term *scaling up* has been used to describe the intentional, guided processes designed to bring proven or promising health care models or practices to more people (Mangham & Hanson, 2010; Ovretveit, 2011; WHO, 2010) and often is used synonymously with *dissemination* and *spread*. Scaling up is any form of expansion of an intervention or approach, not as an end in itself, but as a means to achieve greater and more widespread benefits for the population of concern (Linn, Hartmann, Kharas, Kohl, & Massler, 2010). It signifies urgency, growth, and intention. When new and additional sites or disciplines use a lesson learned or best practice from a PPM integration project, for example, and significant changes to professional practice that go beyond verbalization to include deep processes that change practice and enable better patient outcomes that continue over time, a "shift in ownership" from the original innovator to a new adopter occurs, generating meaningful scale-up (Coburn, 2003).

Scale-up is an active process that aims to benefit more stakeholders and foster institutionalization on a lasting basis. Interest in scale-up has grown in recent years because of the increased urgency to expand successful health care innovations rapidly.

> Raising awareness about lessons learned or best practices during professional practice model integration with the intention of improving implementation or integrating model components better and more widely in new contexts, such that they are embedded in new systems, is more than simply adopting a lesson learned or best practice.

In fact, Management Systems International (MSI; 2012) suggests that testing, clarifying, refining, and simplifying an innovation requires many years of evidence generation. Furthermore, the evidence produced needs to be carefully appraised by those desiring to embrace the innovation. Thus, understanding the type of evidence that exists is essential. For example, the difference between anecdotal reports in one setting and valid and reliable quantitative evidence from several sites in different settings is quite substantial.

Prior to scaling-up activities, evaluating the innovation, lessons learned, or best practices for several characteristics that might demonstrate the best chances for adoption by others has been advocated. They are as follows (WHO, 2010, p. 19):

- Credibility: Is there sound evidence or application by respected persons or institutions?
- Observability: Can potential users see the results in practice?
- Relevance: Are the lessons learned or best practices pertinent to PPM integration issues?
- Advantage: Is there a relative benefit over existing approaches?
- Simplicity: Is it easy to transfer and adopt?

- Compatibility: Do the lessons learned or best practices fit with existing users' established values, norms, and facilities?
- Trialability: Are the lessons learned or best practices able to be tested or tried without committing the potential user to complete the adoption?

In addition, the Scalability Assessment Tool (SAT) checklist (MSI, 2012) containing 28 items is intended to stimulate dialogue and aid in decision making about scale-up activities to facilitate simplifying the scaling-up process. Once the potential viability of an innovation and its evidence base is better known, specific scale-up strategies have been documented that may facilitate the process.

In the WHO document, *Nine Steps for Developing a Scaling-up Strategy* (2010), several approaches for scaling up were identified: vertically (through administrative structural and policy changes), horizontally (extended geographically), functionally (adding on to an existing model), and spontaneously (scaling up without intension or naturally). In practice, these approaches often work together. For example, horizontal and functional scaling up are most likely to succeed when accompanied by vertical scaling up. Although spontaneous scaling up occurs infrequently, guided approaches, involving deliberate efforts to put a best practice or new innovation in place, help ensure that the key elements of the innovation and the context that are needed for success remain in place (Massoud, Donohue, & McCannon, 2010).

Much of what is known about scaling up comes from the international health literature on improving health services in low-income countries. Limited evidence exists for scaling-up lessons learned or best practices, particularly from integration or demonstration projects, including PPMs. Thus, there is no single best approach that can be applied, and most approaches require tailoring to the local situation. Nevertheless, there are a variety of frameworks and methods of distribution that have been reported that may facilitate the way clinicians and leaders approach dissemination.

FRAMEWORKS AND METHODS OF DISTRIBUTION

Dissemination Frameworks

Several frameworks exist for understanding dissemination and spread (Wilson, Petticrew, Calnan, & Nazareth, 2010), but only a select few will be described here. Because effective dissemination entails active strategies for reaching a wide audience, frameworks that use more passive or natural forms of spread will not be included. For example, Rogers's Diffusion of

Innovations Theory (1995; see also Chapter 8) focuses on how, why, and at what rate practices or innovations spread through defined populations and does not specifically describe active dissemination processes or outcomes. And in Malcolm Gladwell's *Tipping Point* (2000), spread is viewed as a natural process that begins with a few people, a "sticky" change or innovation, and a specific context (see also Chapter 8). It does not offer specific strategies for spread or describe methods of application. A number of more active frameworks were found in the health care literature that may offer promising insights and strategies.

The Institute for Healthcare Improvement's (IHI) evolving framework for spread (Massoud, Nielsen, Nolan, Schall, & Sevin, 2006) considers dissemination a leadership responsibility and lists several key issues necessary for successful dissemination. They are as follows (Massoud et al., 2006):

- Preparing for spread
- Establishing an aim for spread
- Developing an initial spread plan
- Establishing and refining the spread plan

This framework has been used in several IHI learning collaboratives such as the 100,000 lives campaign, the Kaiser Permanente system, the End Stage Renal Disease Network, and the California Improvement Network. It has been refined over several years and, because it involves planning and consideration during implementation processes, it is dependent on senior leadership for its success.

The University of Washington Health Promotion Research Center (HPRC) framework (Harris et al., 2012) uses social marketing principles in a practical way to encourage dissemination of research findings to real-world practice environments. It contains two key elements: the resources for disseminating evidence-based practices, which include collaborating researchers and disseminating organizations, and the user organizations that adopt and implement the practice. It requires linking to and learning from the user organization (which has fixed characteristics) to develop relevant and effective dissemination. Although referring to research, it has implications for spreading lessons learned and best practices as well.

The Value-Added Research Dissemination Framework (Macoubrie & Harrison, 2013) was developed for the Administration for Children and Families, U.S. Department of Health and Human Services, after conducting a multidisciplinary (human services, communication, and organization studies) literature review and contains six elements. The core challenges, or the persistent issues that face disseminators, lie at the heart of the framework. The challenges arising from organizations and the disseminator's role, which is to perform or guide a series of activities that address the core challenges, are highlighted and include communication concepts and utilization issues. The framework represents a functional approach to dissemination, and shows four phases: planning, translation and packaging, strategic distribution, and follow through. The Value-Added Research Dissemination Framework emphasizes the disseminator's role in overcoming common dissemination challenges and includes dissemination as a strategic communication process, incorporating concepts from the communication field. The framework considers the complex structure of clinical practice in the United States, strengthening the understanding of challenges inherent in dissemination and offers several solutions. Used to guide dissemination of lessons learned and best practices from professional practice integration, this framework is comprehensive and practical while emphasizing the disseminator's role.

The Dissemination and Implementation Framework (Esposito et al., 2015) was created to enhance awareness and knowledge of useful and relevant information to help people and organizations make decisions and put them into everyday practice. To generate that information, engaging stakeholders as partners from the very beginning of a project is deemed relevant to helping target audiences make real-world choices, potentially improving the likelihood of rapid practice changes. The focus on the engagement of individuals, communities, and organizations is unique and placed at the core of this framework, enabling it to allow those using the framework to better understand the needs of audiences who will use evidence to make health care decisions. Project findings are disseminated to the practice environment where they are applied and evaluated in an iterative process that continues to inform future innovations. Little evidence exists for the effectiveness of this framework as it is relatively novel.

The ExpandNet/WHO framework for scaling up (WHO, 2010) offers a systematic way to consider scale-up guided by four key principles: systems thinking; a focus on sustainability; the need to determine scalability; and respect for gender, equity, and human rights principles. In this holistic framework, five elements (the innovation, the resource team, the user organization, the environment, and the scale-up strategy) are centered and four strategic choice areas (dissemination and advocacy, costs/resource mobilization, monitoring and evaluation, and organizational processes) are provided. The framework, created for underdeveloped nations, is considered a learning process, and changing the strategic plan as learning proceeds is constructive and necessary. Moreover, because learning requires systematic use of evidence, it is essential that data are linked to decision making. Balancing the broad range of factors for scaling up carries out what is desirable and feasible.

In summary, several frameworks exist for reflecting on, learning about, and strategizing for dissemination, spread, and scaling up of lessons learned and best practices related to PPM integration. Common themes among them include: planning dissemination into the integration project at the beginning; consideration of context; responsibility, particularly among leaders; and systematic, active strategies that maximize extension and expansion.

Methods of Distribution

Distribution includes creating networks or conduits in order to spread knowledge gained from research findings or, in this case, lessons learned and best practices resulting from the integration of a PPM, to the widest possible audience. Two primary channels, namely, direct and indirect, act in concert with various subchannels or intermediaries to transfer ideas and materials learned from integrating a PPM at one location to a wider range of existing or potential stakeholders. Distribution involves initial notification, periodic and end-of-project exposure of lessons learned and/or best practices, and ongoing communication of model components to different contexts with the goal of extension and expansion.

> Using clearly articulated channels of communications between the original project personnel and the broader health care recipient, nursing, and health system community, lessons learned and best practices facilitate the perception by additional stakeholders that integrating a professional practice model in a certain manner would advantage them in some way.

In terms of lessons learned and best practices, the goal of distribution is to provide convenient and appropriate mechanisms for facilitating knowledge about them, such that additional users have access to the latest, most effective ideas and approaches. In other words, distribution includes the free flow of information about PPM integration with the intention to influence external stakeholders.

The practical experience and guidance emerging from professional practice model integration at one site is of great value to many potential stakeholders across different sectors and even internationally. It is a leadership responsibility that, when done effectively, differentiates a health system's services and may even lead to an improved identity and influence (reach; brand).

The strategies for distributing lessons learned and best practices include traditional forms of written communications, such as newsletters, publications, and presentations at professional conferences, to more interactive forums such as stakeholder focus groups, websites, videos, and partnerships. Publications and conference materials can span the whole integration experience, including specific methodologies for evaluation, innovative educational instructional materials, effective and efficient feedback mechanisms, information about outcomes, policies developed, or even reflections about certain implementation processes.

Although little research has provided evidence about best distribution approaches, some literature is available for consideration. For example, distribution methods should consider (Reardon, Lavis, & Gibson, 2007):

- The message—is it positive, practical, and tangible?
- The intended audience—what are their characteristics?
- The messenger—is he or she credible?
- The transfer method—is it passive or active?
- The expected outcome—what impact is intended?

Obviously, a message driven by facts or data, is actionable, and the idea that it provokes reflection is appealing. It also helps to deliver the message using a credible messenger (e.g., a peered-reviewed publication, a face-to-face lecture by an expert, or a conversation with a stakeholder who experienced the lessons learned or best practice). Targeting an audience by learning its characteristics and establishing quality relationships built on ongoing exchanges of information and ideas facilitates application. Taking into account the impact of a proposed change on decision makers also improves the chance the message will be heard. For example, considering the resources or expertise required and their availability in certain settings may prompt adapting lessons learned or best practices for specific audiences. Finally, suggesting expected impacts of the lessons learned or best practices, even if results are not yet available, helps determine the scope and potential value of a given course of action.

For example, do the lessons learned or best practices suggest a change in attitudes or awareness, a change in behaviors or policies, or validate the PPM already chosen?

Supporting others by offering tools for assessing these outcomes so that they can monitor results, offering firsthand visits or conference calls, and maintain ongoing collaborative relationships promotes the lessons learned or best practices as enabling integration strategies.

More recent, McNichol and Grimshaw (2014) emphasized patient or stakeholder involvement in distribution so that the message reaches stakeholders early and often. In relation to PPM integration, employing this approach requires early and ongoing robust relationships with patients and families, nurses, and other health systems.

Using appropriate language, listening to what is important, and involving stakeholders with implementation and evaluation strategies, authorship, and choosing dissemination strategies ensures relevancy to the intended recipient and provides important input to the ongoing evolution of professional practice model components, possibly speeding up decisions and expanded future applications.

This approach is aligned with PCORI's Dissemination and Implementation Framework (Esposito et al., 2015), which focuses on stakeholder engagement and fits with many nursing theories.

LEADERSHIP AND DISSEMINATION

The frameworks reviewed stressed planning for dissemination at the beginning of PPM integration versus at the end, and incorporating the planned strategies in the implementation process. A thoughtful dissemination plan allows health systems to move beyond the simple listing of lessons learned and best practices; rather, it uses a variety of means to reach any and all designated target audiences.

As leaders of a professional practice, nurses (and nurse leaders) have a responsibility to convey lessons learned and best practices from professional practice model integration experiences to others in order to expedite the intended outcomes to a wider range of stakeholders.

The following action steps may facilitate dissemination:

- Determine and document the goals of dissemination as they relate to lessons learned and best practices; include in project implementation.
- Clarify in specific behavioral terms the objectives of dissemination; include in project implementation.
- Reflect on the scope and characteristics of "potential users" that dissemination activities are designed to reach for each objective; describe the capabilities and resources that will be required to access the content.
- Identify the basic elements of the potential lessons learned and best practices that need to be disseminated to each of the potential user groups identified.
- Identify the primary source or sources that each potential user group is already tied into or most respects; use these sources in the dissemination approaches.
- Describe the medium or media through which the content of dissemination messages can best be delivered to potential users.
- Describe how dissemination activities will be considered successful (i.e. identify indicators). Hint: If objectives are written in behavioral terms, this will already be established.
- Determine what dissemination data needs to be gathered, its collection, frequency of collection, responsibility for gathering and analyzing data, and communicating results; add to PPM integration evaluation plan.
- Identify access to lessons learned and best practice information and how it will be archived for later use. Consider that others will use project-related information when they perceive a need for it—not necessarily when the project is completed.
- Develop strategies for promoting awareness of the availability of lessons learned and best practice information in multiple formats.
- Identify potential barriers that may interfere with the targeted users' access or utilization of dissemination materials; develop actions to reduce these barriers.

For example, barriers to access of lessons learned and best practices may exist in the following areas:

- Potential users are not ready for the change.
- The format and level of information needed is greater than anticipated.
- There is a lack of clear relevance to others' needs.

- The context is greatly different, requiring alternate forms of communication.
- Only certain information sources are trusted.

Negative perceptions of the messenger, such as limited credibility, suspicions concerning motives or lack of sensitivity to users' concerns, may impede adoption of lessons learned or best practices because they generate uncertainty in the potential user. Uncertainty creates anxiety, doubt, or even perceived threats, hindering potential users' perceived usefulness or relevance of a certain innovation. When lessons learned are not considered relevant or the evidence presented is not valid and reliable, resulting in doubt about its trustworthiness, and easier approaches are available, health systems will naturally make alternative decisions about application in their sites. Finally, costs and resources required are prohibitive in many contexts today, making it crucial to address these needs up front.

On the other hand, using a grounded theory approach with elders in four home care organizations that had implemented best practices in Canada, Ploeg et al. (2014) found three factors that facilitated spread processes. Based on interviews conducted with front-line providers, managers, and directors at baseline ($n = 44$) and 1 year later ($n = 40$), leading with passion and commitment, sustaining strategies, and seeing the benefits were identified as spread facilitators. Leaders were seen as driving forces for spread, particularly their ability to develop trusting and respectful relationships with front-line providers. Ongoing engagement, communication, coaching, and evaluation feedback helped to sustain best practices across systems, and the benefits realized were crucial, particularly those that impacted patients and families. The critical role of leaders at multiple levels was consistent with other studies of spread.

> To reduce the gap between lessons learned and best practices identified at one site to many and different health care sites, nurses and nurse leaders must take the dissemination/spread/scale-up phase of integration as seriously as implementation.

Creating a professional culture of practice that differs from what was used in the past is underpinned by nursing theory and is fueled by science; it requires planning dissemination activities into the integration process so that others choose to use and evaluate them in their own sites, benefitting a wider range of stakeholders.

By clarifying tangible, effective, and efficient approaches to professional practice model integration, describing the processes used, and with sensitivity to messages extended, nurses and nurse leaders may accelerate the proliferation of professional practice models in health systems, ultimately benefitting patients, other nurses, the discipline, and health systems.

Ensuring that colleagues receive, read, understand, and appreciate the value of a certain approach and then fostering the use of it in their own institution is a necessary implementation strategy.

In addition to traditional media, human networks, such as learning communities, partnerships, research networks, discussion boards, journal clubs, consultation, local media presentations, and other forms of active, engaging, and face-to-face strategies are needed. For example, a team-based research network in one study facilitated the rapid collection of a large data set and adoption of best practices (Puga, Stevens, & Patel, 2013). Advocating for policy changes that facilitate more widespread use of lessons learned and best practices both locally and through professional associations often engages multiple and varied professionals in interactive dialogue. The need for future research to evaluate the impact of human, interactive dissemination approaches of lessons learned and best practices is great; however, nurses and nurse leaders can stimulate such activities by ensuring that dissemination is a prominent component of PPM integration project planning.

SUMMARY

This chapter provided an overview of disseminating lessons learned and best practices identified as a result of integrating a PPM. Lessons learned and best practices were defined with the ultimate goal of application in additional sites and contexts in order to benefit additional patients, families, nurses, and health systems—stakeholders of PPMs. Frameworks and strategies for dissemination were explained with special emphasis on those active, health care-oriented approaches that extend or expand relevant lessons learned and best practices. The term *scaling up* was described, including specific scale-up strategies. Direct and indirect methods of distribution were explained with attention to the message, the messenger, the audience, the transfer methods, and the outcomes of dissemination. Finally, the role of nurses and nursing leadership in terms of generating and following a dissemination plan and using traditional and more contemporary interactive approaches to effectively spread lessons learned and best practice was advanced.

REFLECTIVE APPLICATIONS

For Students

1. Explain the importance of sharing lessons learned and best practices. Whose responsibility is it? How is this best accomplished?
2. Differentiate between the terms *lessons learned* and *best practices*. Why is this important? Provide an example of each. How might these affect your attitudes or behavior?
3. Why is the dissemination process so prolonged? Explain how nurses and nurse leaders have contributed to this? What could be done to lessen the time required for dissemination, particularly concerning PPM integration?
4. Define the term *scaling up*. What have we learned from international health care projects that informs our understanding of scale-up? Provide references for your examples.
5. Choose one dissemination framework discussed in this chapter. Evaluate it for clarity, usefulness, comprehensiveness, evidence demonstrated, and overall strengths and weaknesses. How might it be used by those on the verge of integrating a PPM? Please explain.
6. Develop a lesson learned or best practice and identify a distribution method for it. Describe its message, the messenger, the audience, transfer methods, and potential outcomes. How would you predict it would be received by others?
7. Discuss how you can best prepare for dissemination activities in your future career.
8. Describe how nurses can improve dissemination of lessons learned and best practices. Provide two examples. What are their outcomes? How could you work together with the nurse leader to ensure effectively and timely dissemination of lessons learned or best practices?

For Clinical Nurses

1. Discuss why dissemination of lessons learned and best practices related to PPM integration is important. Provide an example of how it might benefit other nurses.
2. Analyze whether dissemination practices at your health system are effective and efficient. Discuss how direct care nurses are involved. Be specific and provide examples.
3. How does the leadership team at your health system ensure scale-up of new programs internally and externally? How do you know? Based on the knowledge you acquired from reading this chapter, what could be done differently to better facilitate scale-up?

4. Think about your unit. What lessons learned and/or best practices were . identified during the past year? How do they inform practice at other sites? Were they effectively and efficiently disseminated? What distribution methods were used? If none were identified, why not? What can you do to facilitate more efficient identification of lessons learned or best practices?

5. Suggest three ideas that you could use to promote dissemination of lessons learned or best practices based on the PPM at your institution. How could you get coworkers or leaders involved?

6. Name at least two ways you could expand your skills in dissemination. Now, create a plan to develop these skills and hold yourself accountable for that achievement.

For Nurse Leaders

1. Who in your organization is responsible for disseminating lessons learned and best practices related to PPM integration? How has this been accomplished? Quantify the successes.

2. What traditional or nontraditional forms of distribution are typically used in your health system to disseminate information? Be specific.

3. Discus the statement "ensuring that colleagues receive, read, understand, and appreciate the value of a certain approach and then fostering the use of it in their own institution is a necessary implementation strategy" (p. 248). What does this mean to you? How does nursing leadership meet its responsibility regarding dissemination of lessons learned and best practices?

4. How could accessing lessons learned and best practices about PPM integration help you and your health system? Explain how a nurse leader can promote using such information prior to or during PPM integration? What would he or she have to do?

5. What forums exist in your health system to help nurse leaders or direct care nurses reflect on their experiences so that lessons learned and best practices can be identified and clarified? How could you facilitate these? What limitations exist? Can you identify someone in the organization whom you could work with on this?

6. Explain the difference between lessons learned and best practices.

7. What factors would hamper your health system from adopting lessons learned or best practices? Why? Which might facilitate their adoption? Be specific and provide examples of each. What is your role regarding such factors?

8. Provide an example from the last time a program, service, or policy was "scaled up" in your health system. Consider the following scale-up strategies: vertical, horizontal, functional, or spontaneous. What strategy was used in your example? Was it planned? Why or why not? Did it work? How do you know?

9. What dissemination framework from this chapter most resonates with you? Why? How can you incorporate it to improve dissemination of lessons learned and best practices?

10. Describe the distribution methods you use for dissemination. How effective are they? How do you know? How efficient are they? How do you know? How could you revise these to improve dissemination? Or could you? Why?

11. How does stakeholder involvement fit with your thoughts on dissemination? What can you do to increase stakeholder engagement in dissemination?

For Nurse Educators

1. What learning activities could best help undergraduate students apply their professional role in dissemination of findings from health care innovations? Why is this important for them to understand? What about graduate students?

2. What evidence is available to help you best demonstrate effective dissemination? How might this apply to your current curriculum?

3. Develop at least three objectives for a learning activity focused on dissemination. What evaluation methods will you use to ensure its comprehension and application?

4. Develop a learning activity using "the message, the messenger, the audience, the transfer method, and the intended outcomes" (p. 248) to help students learn about dissemination. In what program or level do you see its relevance? How could this learning activity be revised for nurse leaders?

5. How are patients and families used in your curriculum to advance learning? How might they be? How would involving patients and families enhance or limit current faculty behavior? Be specific. How could you help facilitate patient and family involvement in student learning? What about their participation in learning dissemination concepts?

6. What specific experiences would help students learn to differentiate lessons learned and best practices? How might these be used by faculty to enhance students' learning?

7. What lessons learned and best practices are generated by your programs? Are they effective and efficient? Through what distribution channels are they disseminated? How do you personally enact your responsibility for dissemination?
8. How often does your school or program adopt lessons learned or best practices? Why?
9. Describe the "scale-up" of a recent new program at your educational institution. What strategy was used in your example? Was it planned? Why or why not? Did it work? How do you know? Based on the knowledge you acquired from reading this chapter, what could be done differently to better facilitate scale-up?

LEARNING FROM THE FIELD: AN INTERVIEW WITH TWO VICE PRESIDENTS ON "SCALING UP"

Background

Advocate Health is the largest integrated health care delivery system in Illinois, consisting of 11 acute care hospitals, one children's hospital (two campuses), and over 250 sites of care. In 2013, Advocate Health Care responded to its commitment to nursing by hiring the first ever system chief nurse executive. This new leader is focused on building a solid infrastructure to support key areas of nursing: business operations, clinical informatics, clinical development and education, and nursing practice.

In the spring of 2014, nurses from across the system gathered for a daylong advocate nursing summit. Sixty percent of participants were direct care nurses and the remainder included nurses in education, advanced practice, and leadership roles. The agenda included detailing the characteristics of the advocate nurse, designing a PPM representative of nursing across the enterprise, including selection of a nurse theorist. The resulting PPM was believed to provide the foundation for nurses to advance the practice of nursing and enhance relationships with those they serve, which strongly supported the system's mission.

In planning for the implementation of this model, it became evident that the underlying theoretical framework provided the common ground needed to emphasize the balance between clinical or disease-driven care and a more patient-centered focus. Additionally, the framework was tapped for its ability to move toward a system-wide approach.

As internal and external forces necessitate change at a very fast pace, the integration of our PPM proved to be an exciting and challenging time for nursing at Advocate Health. The resiliency and adaptability of nurses were and remain essential to best prepare us for the future.

Interview

Question: Have you identified any lessons learned or best practices during this past year as you attempted to spread the PPM across the system?

Response: A key lesson learned was identified as the need to engage leaders at each site to assist with application. With multiple campuses, there was much variability in leader engagement and some control issues as you might expect. Such assistance needs to be consistent in terms of the actual message, and also in how it is conveyed. For example, the individual site "voice" should describe essential practice elements, defined consistently so that the foundation for practice remains non-negotiable throughout the system. However, at the same time, it is recognized that individual sites have unique cultures and patient populations, so it is also necessary to honor these by allowing some variation. Thus, we tried to gain the individual chief nurse executive's high level of conceptual agreement while allowing some reasonable tolerance (related to specific details) for variation at each site.

Question: Did you design dissemination into your implementation plan?

Response: To tell you the truth, not consciously! Although we always thought about the whole system, the necessary elements of dissemination, including dissemination goals, were not documented. It is a work in progress. If we had to do it all over again, we would do if differently— perhaps use a different communication approach, more systematic and coordinated methods, and connect our work outside of the nursing department. We have plans for publication and presentation, but no specifics.

Question: What forums exist to help the system reflect on its experiences so that lessons learned and best practices can be identified and further developed?

Response: Our existing leadership meetings, educational and Magnet®-related meetings, and the annual summit could be used for this purpose, if we set aside some designated time.

Question: What distribution strategies did you use at the various sites?

Response: We used the typical educational strategies, such as PowerPoints and flyers, but we could have communicated better through more frequent e-mails and other forms of communication. We also allowed leaders some creativity in developing processes, such as talking points. We tried to maintain system cohesiveness while leveraging site strengths and defining characteristics.

Question: If you had to do it all over again, what would you do differently with respect to dissemination across the system?

Response: Redesign education—work more collegially—taking turns. We have redesigned our educational programs and they are now housed in regions versus at individual sites or centrally. We think this will help spread the model. Another point is to remain aware that at individual sites, the question—How does this impact *my* site?—is the predominant thought. At the central office, we need to remind ourselves of that often.

Alice Siehoff
Susan Okuno-Jones

REFERENCES

Best practices. (2015). Retrieved from http://www.businessdictionary.com/definition/best-practice.html

Coburn, C. (2003). Rethinking scale: Moving beyond numbers to deep and lasting change. *Educational Researcher, 32*(6), 3–12.

Colquhoun, A., Aplin, L., Geary, J., Goodman, K. J., & Hatcher, J. (2012). Challenges created by data dissemination and access restrictions when attempting to address community concerns: Individual privacy versus public wellbeing. *International Journal of Circumpolar Health, 71*, 1–7. doi:10.3402/ijch.v71i0.18414

Esposito, D., Heeringa, J., Bradley, K., Croake, S., & Kimmey, L (2015). *PCORI dissemination and implementation framework*. Washington, DC: Patient-Centered Outcomes Research Institute. Retrieved from http://www.mathematica-mpr.com/~/media/publications/pdfs/health/pcori%20di%20framework%20draft.pdf

Gladwell, M. (2002). *The tipping point: How little things can make a big difference*. New York, NY: Little, Brown, and Company.

Glasgow, R. E., Vinson, C., Chambers, D., Khoury, M. J., Kaplan, R. M., & Hunter, C. (2012). National Institutes of Health approaches to dissemination and implementation science: Current and future directions. *American Journal of Public Health, 102*(7), 1274–1281.

Greenhalgh, T., Robert, G., MacFarlane, F., Bate, P., & Kyriakidou, O. (2004). Diffusion of innovations in service organizations: Systematic review and recommendations. *Milbank Quarterly, 82*(4), 581–629.

Harris, J. R., Cheadle, A., Hannon, P. A., Forehand, M., Lichiello, P., Mahoney, E., . . . Yarrow, J. (2012). A framework for disseminating evidence-based health promotion practices. *Preventing Chronic Disease, 9*. 110081. doi:10.5888/pcd9.110081

Linn, J. F., Hartmann, A., Kharas, H., Kohl, R., & Massler, B. (2010). Scaling up the fight against rural poverty. *Brookings Institution: Global Economy and Development.* Retrieved from http://www.brookings.edu/~/media/research/files/papers/2010/10/ifad-linn-kharas/10_ifad_linn_kharas.pdf

Macoubrie, J., & Harrison, C. (2013). *The value-added research dissemination framework* (Office of Planning Research and Evaluation report #2013–10). Washington, DC: Office of Planning, Research and Evaluation, Administration for Children and Families, U. S. Department of Health and Human Services. Retrieved March 26, 2015, from http://www.acf.hhs.gov/sites/default/files/opre/valueadded.pdf

Management Systems International (MSI). (2012). *Scaling up—From vision to large-scale change: A management framework for practitioners* (2nd ed.). Washington, DC: Author. Retrieved March 30, 2015, from http://www.acf.hhs.gov/sites/default/files/opre/valueadded.pdf

Mangham, L. J., & Hanson, K. (2010). Scaling up in international health: What are the key issues? *Health Policy and Planning, 25*(2), 85–96.

Massoud, M. R., Donohue, K. L., & McCannon, C. J. (2010). Options for large-scale spread of simple, high-impact interventions: Technical report. *USAID Health Care Improvement Project.* Retrieved January 19, 2014, from http://www.fgcasal.org/aeets/Documentos/MassoudDonahueMcCannonLargeScaleSpreadHighImpactInterventions_USAIDURCSept10.pdf

Massoud, M. R., Nielsen, G. A., Nolan, K., Schall, M. W., & Sevin, C. (2006). *A framework for spread: From local improvements to system-wide change* (Institute for Healthcare Improvement Innovation Series white paper). Cambridge, MA: Institute for Healthcare Improvement.

McNichol, E., & Grimshaw, P. (2014). An innovative toolkit: Increasing the role and value of patient and public involvement in the dissemination of research findings. *International Practice Development Journal, 4*(1), 1–14.

Ovretveit, J. (2011). Widespread focused improvement: Lessons from international health for spreading specific improvements to health services in high-income countries. *International Journal for Quality in Health Care, 23*(3), 239–246.

Ploeg, J., Markle-Reid, M., Davies, B., Higuchi, K., Gifford, W., Bajnok, I., . . . Bookey-Bassett, S. (2014). Spreading and sustaining best practices for home care of older adults: A grounded theory study. *Implementation Science, 9,* 162. doi:10.1186/s13012-014-0162-4

Puga, F., Stevens, K. R., & Patel, D. I. (2013). Adopting best practices from team science in a healthcare improvement research network: The impact on dissemination and implementation. *Nursing Research and Practice, 2013,* 1–7. doi:10.1155/2013/814360

Reardon, R., Lavis, J., & Gibson, J. (2007). *From research to practice: A knowledge transfer planning guide.* Toronto, ON, Canada: Institute for Work & Health.

Rogers, E. M. (1995). *Diffusion of innovations.* New York, NY: Free Press.

Wilson, P. M., Petticrew, M., Calnan, M. W., & Nazareth, I. (2010). Disseminating research findings: What should researchers do? A systematic scoping review of conceptual frameworks. *Implementation Science, 5,* 91. doi:10.1186/1748-5908-5-91

World Health Organization (WHO). (2008). *Guide for documenting and sharing best practices in health programs.* Brazzaville, Republic of Congo: Author.

World Health Organization (WHO). (2010). *Nine steps for developing a scaling-up strategy.* Geneva, Switzerland: Author. Retrieved January 21, 2014, from http://www.fgcasal.org/aeets/Documentos/MassoudDonahueMcCannonLarge-ScaleSpreadHighImpactInterventions_USAIDURCSept10.pdf

CHAPTER	12

Power of Professional Practice Models: Impact

KEY WORDS

Impact, future, value, partnerships, networks, learning communities

OBJECTIVES

By the end of this chapter, readers will be able to:

1. Describe the potential impact of professional practice models (PPMs)
2. Discriminate between the terms *dissemination* and *impact*
3. Evaluate the types of impact
4. Describe three methods used to link value-based outputs with others
5. Differentiate among partnerships, networks, and learning communities
6. Identify at least three sources of external information that can facilitate future planning

IMPACT OF PROFESSIONAL PRACTICE MODELS

For health systems, integrating professional practice models (PPMs) simultaneously carries with it risk and opportunity. For instance, the effort requires tremendous investment of resources and, if it fails, the investment could be wasted, a huge risk for most health systems. On the other hand, the opportunities for expediting the implementation, improving nursing practice, and/or positively influencing patient outcomes may exceed intended outcomes and have significant utility for others if the PPMs are translated into real-world solutions. For example, employee passion for a particular PPM component, a successful and efficient approach to implementation, popular training strategies, valid and reliable evaluation methods, or improved patient outcomes might yield practical dividends that have implications for populations, professional practice, resource consumption, policy, teaching, and knowledge advancement. In fact, PPM integration at one site is not necessarily an end in itself; rather, positive consequences can generate significant value at many locations. New ways of practicing nursing, innovative indications for existing nursing practice, cost savings, advancements in knowledge, increases in employee work engagement, revised policies, and important and improved patient outcomes are examples of noticeable outcomes that provide evidence of impact.

Impact refers to the effect or consequence of an innovation (e.g., a PPM) or research findings that makes a difference in the real world (versus academia), implying that actions or activities that lead to some change are involved (Chandler, 2014). For instance, if an innovation has been successfully demonstrated in one site and is used by practitioners in another site leading to similar improvements, its impact may be viewed as effective. However, if additional organizations take up the innovation or if the degree of improvements is greater than originally demonstrated, the innovation is considered to have a powerful impact.

Although most of the literature on impact refers to the results of research, the investment of time and resources required to integrate large-scale change, as intended by PPM integration, demands consideration.

Because health care expenditures continue to rise and reimbursement policies have changed, monetary resources remain limited and accountability for large investments has become a major leadership responsibility. Thus, demonstrating the value of PPM integration through the eyes of stakeholders at all levels requires leaders to adjust results reporting from gut feelings or activities completed to providing real evidence of value (evidence-based leadership). Such evidence also is a necessary antecedent to others' utilization of demonstrated successes.

For example, using or citing a reference to an innovation from a peer-reviewed journal suggests that it is perceived by others in the field as having an influence on the field and/or society as a whole and may benefit additional organizations or populations. Or, adopting a well-demonstrated theoretical framework at multiple sites, and then disseminating it through an annual system-wide leadership conference points to impact. Using evidence from PPM integration in this way may accelerate benefits and create opportunity for others and the profession.

THE NATURE OF IMPACT

Impact shifts what is learned through innovation (or research) at one site to actionable recommendations and applications of such knowledge in a variety of practice settings and contexts. It is similar to the research term *knowledge translation*, which has been defined as: "the synthesis, exchange, and application of knowledge by relevant stakeholders to accelerate the benefits of global and local innovation in strengthening health systems and improving people's health" (Pablos-Mendez & Shademani, 2006, p. 82), with the ultimate goal of enabling and reinforcing change on a larger scale. Furthermore, impact is an interactive process reinforced by ongoing exchanges between the original innovators who created the knowledge (lessons learned and best practices) and those who use it.

The Payback Framework (Buxton & Hanney, 1996), a widely used model for assessing the impact of research, suggested that awareness and new knowledge, better informed research, policy recommendations, commercial product development, adoption of the innovation by practitioners and the public, improved health, cost reduction, and other economic benefits were "paybacks" from the research process. The United Kingdom's Economic and Social Research Council (2015) classifies impact as:

- Instrumental: Influencing the development of policy, practice, or service provision, shaping legislation, altering behavior
- Conceptual: Contributing to the understanding of policy issues, reframing debates
- Capacity building: Technical and personal skill development

A similar way of imagining the benefits from investments of health systems toward integrating PPMs can be offered. Because most health systems receive public resources and have missions that "serve society" (albeit locally), successful evidence from large-scale projects demonstrates to governments, stakeholders, and the wider public, the value (impact) of such projects. Furthermore, as nurses, our contract with society includes facilitating the progress between what is known and what is practiced, spending resources wisely in the process.

To ensure that innovation investments are spent most effectively and remain a priority in the face of limited resources, it is essential that nurses and nurse leaders obtain the most reliable estimates of the value of innovation investments.

From the patient's view, value may include access to services, quality of those services (including safety and outcomes), and perceptions about the experiences. However, in the eyes of top-level administration, tangible (e.g., reduced costs resulting from shorter lengths of stay, reduced nurse turnover) and intangible measures (e.g., employee teamwork, corporate image) are used together to create a monetary profile that demonstrates how an organization benefitted from an innovation. Responsible use of health systems' funds demands balanced and credible evidence that demonstrates benefit to the system (e.g., better market share, reduced costs, increased brand awareness) to stimulate others' use, the real meaning of impact. The process of demonstrating monetary value (of PPM integration)—return on investment (ROI)—is a systematic process that is related closely to the evaluation plan (in other words, the data inputs, objective measurement, and results). The ROI can then be calculated as a percentage: earnings divided by investments or the net benefits in dollars (project benefits minus the costs) times 100 (Buzachero, Phillips, Phillips, & Phillips, 2013). Communicating these results to various stakeholders helps convince them that the system's resources were wisely spent and helps ensure the project's continuance.

Often, nurses and nurse leaders fail to see that the financial success of a large-scale project, such as PPM integration, is their responsibility.

> Carefully aligning and realigning (over time) PPM integration with important health system business goals is necessary to drive perceived value.

For example, in the early developmental period, cautiously choosing evaluation metrics that align with corporate measures of performance (e.g., patient experience, employee engagement, reduced errors, patient wait times, unplanned readmissions) establishes a fundamental link to business goals.

> Anticipating how to translate intended changes in patient or nurse outcomes to dollar values ensures a more efficient reporting process.

Realizing that external and contextual factors can influence the agreed-on outcomes measures, nurses and nurse leaders should clarify these ahead of time and use them to interpret and explain results. Working effectively with key leaders in other departments (e.g., the financial department, decision support), and insisting on their ongoing support, is also needed to contribute to project success.

The impact of PPM integration on a health system and beyond varies as the project adheres (or not) to the original values and implementation strategies, and adapts based on experiences and improvements used, suggesting that *levels* of impact may be observed.

> Identifying how key stakeholders will benefit from the knowledge obtained in an integration project, by categorizing the evidence gained into system or practice groups, creating opportunities to interact with them (through various dissemination activities), and providing practice guidance may increase the extent of impact.

The number of successfully demonstrated and documented lessons learned/best practices that are cited by others; the number of sites and contexts in which knowledge from an integration project is used; the number of patients affected; the copyrights or licenses developed; the number of policies informed or developed; the number of sites where new work processes become institutionalized; and the new capacities of employees affected are just a few examples of the extent of impact (level, range, or scope). Capturing these outputs adds to the evidence base needed to demonstrate value and is powerful in terms of persuading others. Documenting and advancing such degrees of impact, along with identifying enablers, is a leadership responsibility.

CREATING HIGH-IMPACT CONNECTIONS

The ability to rapidly mobilize knowledge is central to transforming professional nursing practice and positively impacting patient outcomes. But it is generally not sufficient to merely be aware of and/or access relevant knowledge because many studies have demonstrated the long time lag between available evidence and its uptake in practice (Williamson, Almaskari, Lester, & Maguire, 2015). Rather, to effectively and rapidly influence others, the information (or content) must be understood and match user needs, various communication strategies must be used, and stakeholders must engage in the new innovation and effectively *apply* it, all prerequisites to extending reach (Woolf et al., 2015).

Knowledge translation is a contextual, interactive process that is often complex and dependent on relationships for its effectiveness and efficiency. Baumbusch et al. (2008), referring to research, conceptualizes this "as a dialogic, collaborative engagement between researchers and practitioners through which people come to reflect on what they do, and its consequences, and identify what they might do differently" (p. 134). However, the knowledge generated as a result of integrating a PPM has many implications for others that, if not incorporated efficiently, contributes to significant delays in its uptake in additional health systems. Thus, actively engaging in ways to link value-based outputs with others is a professional responsibility.

> Respecting the context of others, including their unique needs, helping to translate outcomes derived at one site into practical solutions at their sites, and establishing collaborative forums for dialogue facilitate this process. Likewise, respecting the outputs identified by original users, actively listening to their perspectives, choosing to "see" the relevance of such knowledge and apply it in different settings, all in the context of mutually beneficial relationships, facilitate more widespread application.

Various methods and forums that ease the transfer of knowledge gained from one site to others already exist, whereas others are emerging. For example, existing written approaches, such as the literature, professional conferences, websites, published toolkits, and case studies, make a wide variety of new knowledge available to others. But more active approaches, such as partnerships, interactive workshops, learning communities, and collaborative networks, establish the necessary linkage and exchange between knowledge producers and knowledge users to create lasting impact. For example, academic–practice partnerships, defined as strategic relationships between educational and clinical practice settings that are established to advance their mutual interests (AACN, 1990) "are a critical key to strengthen nursing practice and assist nursing in leading change and advancing health care in our communities" (Gale & Beal, 2013, p. 21). Successful benefits in both parties have been reported (Beal, 2012); adopting this model between health systems may yield similar results. Furthermore, research networks are alliances between multiple practice sites that agree to work together to answer common research questions. Unlike traditional research conducted in universities, research networks involve relationships between researchers and clinicians from real-world practices. Similarly, health systems aligned around similar PPMs may use such networks to advance research and evaluation of PPM integration.

Originating in education, professional learning communities include groups of interested professionals (e.g., direct care nurses and nurse leaders) who share common goals and attitudes and who meet regularly over time to collaborate on mutual goals (e.g., accelerating the integration of PPMs; Smith, Shochet, Keeley, Fleming, & Moynahan, 2014). The group uses active techniques to better understand integration such as patient-centered discussions, patient-led seminars, case studies, dialogue with clinical nurses in the real world, site visits, interactive conferences, collaborative projects, pilot studies or demonstration projects, and critical reflection. Through such dynamic and collaborative methods, the necessary give-and-take between various professionals undertaking a similar goal establishes strong and vibrant relationships that are essential in driving application.

In active forums such as these, similar aims are shared, including the desire to understand what works in "real-world" settings.

In relation to integration of PPMs, health systems that share similar models (e.g., use the same theoretical foundation) have logical collective aims; thus, it is natural to join together to examine experiences, share ideas and outcomes, and help each other expedite evidence of their impact.

Another active form of knowledge transfer is the mentorship model. Mentorship is a relational process that is shaped by its structure and leans toward goals (Karcher, Kuperminc, Portwood, Sipe, & Taylor, 2006). It is a voluntary relationship that usually lasts long term. In a systematic review of mentoring as it relates to knowledge translation, Gagliardi et al. (2009) reported that, of the 13 studies eligible for review, all but one reported improvements in knowledge, skill, or behavior. Some barriers to mentoring, such as the need for infrastructure, matching, and training, lack of clarity in mentoring goals, and limited satisfaction with mentors' availability, were noted. Nevertheless, asking a more experienced leader from an institution that has had successfully demonstrated the impact of a PPM for a mentoring opportunity may have benefits for both the mentor and the mentee.

Finally, creating informal forums to directly connect with stakeholders, such as community advisory boards, patient councils, hospital boards, and nursing committees, creates personal connections that are important in establishing credibility and influence. These critical relationships build the trust so necessary for effective decision making and often go untapped in the busyness of integrating PPMs.

In short, creating the connections that rapidly activate knowledge and extend applications of PPMs, including using active exchanges, such as informal and formal arrangements, may help hasten the large-scale change that is so fundamental to demonstrating value.

As Lavis, Robertson, Woodside, McLeod, and Abelson (2003) suggested: "The specifics of a knowledge-transfer strategy must be fine-tuned to the types of decisions [practitioners] face and the types of decision-making environments in which they live" (p. 224). Nurses and nurse leaders may choose from a variety of linkage and exchange approaches or create their own in order to maximize lasting impact.

ACTUALIZING THE FUTURE

In an era of big data, remotely delivered health care; personalized medicine; point-of-care diagnostics; empowered patients; printing of organs; and sophisticated body sensors; all functioning within a culture of social media housed on portable tablets, phones, and watches; the greatest asset of health systems—its nurses—seems intangible. Yet, nurses are key to high-quality patient outcomes (Cheung, Aiken, Clarke, & Sloane, 2008; Kutney-Lee et al., 2009).

> In particular, nurses who appreciate their value, use a disciplinary frame of reference, practice in accord with their values and disciplinary perspective, participate in governance, and are regularly recognized for their performance provide a significant contribution to patients, the discipline, and their health systems.

When combining disciplinary perspectives with program and evaluation methods in a systematic manner, together with various dissemination approaches, nurses and nurse leaders could better position themselves to demonstrate their value. But, adding tactics from the business world, nurses and nurse leaders may be in powerful positions to *lead* new and innovative health systems.

Scanning and monitoring, for example, are types of forecasting used in business in which events and trends in the external environment are noticed and then used to make decisions. In particular, political and economic trends, and also social, technological, and disciplinary trends are examined. Ask questions such as: What do others in similar markets intend to do in the future? How will their activities affect health systems? As a stakeholder, what do these intended activities mean? Scanning helps health systems "see" emerging trends and then, through monitoring those trends, systems are able to detect their meaning. Effective monitoring requires identification of important stakeholders and their needs and the system's reputation among them (nurses know this well).

Various sources exist to gather external information. Some include health care directories, professional journals, newspapers, books, newsletters, government publications, annual reports of health care companies, market research reports, consultants, educational institutions, testing laboratories, social media, advertisements, websites, and through personal acquaintances and professional colleagues who willingly share information. Hence, actively observing and paying attention to novel developments at conferences, regularly reading the literature—including newspapers—scanning others' marketing materials, using knowledgeable consultants with multiple contacts, and networking are important nursing responsibilities. Using such information to build future scenarios, simulations, or to analyze assumptions about the future yields plausible alternatives that may influence health systems' strategic direction.

Scanning, monitoring, and assumption analysis allows nurses and nurse leaders access to important competitive and future-directed disciplinary inclinations, provides commercialization ideas, helps to anticipate risks, and identifies possible alliances and opportunities—information that facilitates the adjustment of current and future practice for maximum advantage, allowing preparation for things to come, and direction for allocation of resources. This guidance positions nursing to *lead* in a health system that is complex and dynamic.

However, leading change or transition requires knowledge and skill that still eludes the discipline. For example, Pittman, Bass, and Hargraves (2015) reported that nurses still only represent about 6% of board members in health systems and leadership training remains limited. The demand for knowledgeable, holistic, team-based nurses who are experts in relationship building and can demonstrate their value through actionable data has never been greater. Continuing to improve the educational levels of all nurses; aligning practice with nursing values and disciplinary frameworks; generating, gathering, and using evidence to improve practice; and sharing leadership and governance will provide the necessary groundwork.

Shaping the future depends on the ability of nurses and nurse leaders to understand their value, assess and document its effect on patient and system outcomes, and link that evidence to tangible real-world outcomes that stakeholders care about.

SUMMARY

This chapter described the nature of impact related to PPM integration, including the definition, types, and associated leadership responsibilities. Impact was discussed as an actionable, interactive process actualized by exchanges between original innovators and those who subsequently choose to apply it. The Payback Framework, a model for assessing research impact, was summarized and categories of impact were explored. ROI, the process for demonstrating the monetary value of PPM integration, was discussed as useful for stakeholder decision making.

Nurses and nurse leaders who rapidly connect with others to affect application in additional sites extend impact. Partnerships, networks, learning communities, mentorship, and informal stakeholder forums were described as possible methods. Finally, using business strategies, such as scanning, monitoring, and analyzing assumptions, helps nurses and nurse leaders anticipate risk and identify possibilities that position them for shaping future health care systems.

REFLECTIVE APPLICATIONS

For Students

1. What health system risks are associated with PPM integration?
2. Explain *impact*. How does it relate to PPM integration? Whose responsibility is it? Why is it important?
3. List some positive consequences of PPM integration that demonstrate impact. Create one of your own.
4. Differentiate between the terms *dissemination* and *impact*. Why is this important? Provide an example of each.
5. Provide an example of a powerful impact from PPM integration. Explain what responsibilities nurses and nurse leaders have in relation to this? What could be done to hasten its application?
6. Look up the Payback Framework. Evaluate it for clarity, usefulness, comprehensiveness, evidence demonstrated, and overall strengths and weaknesses. How might it be used by those integrating a PPM? Please explain.
7. Discuss how you might use the contents of this chapter in the next phase of your future career.

For Clinical Nurses

1. Discuss why the risks and benefits of PPM integration are important for clinical nurses to understand? Provide examples.

2. Analyze whether your health system has "impacted" others particularly in relation to professional nursing practice. Discuss how direct care nurses were involved. Be specific and provide examples.
3. How does the leadership team in your health system ensure that new programs or projects create impact for others? How do you know? Based on the knowledge you acquired from reading this chapter, what could be done differently to better facilitate more widespread application in other sites?
4. Think about the professional practice of nursing on your unit. What are you most proud of? What impact could it have for those in other departments? What about individuals external to the organization? How do you ensure that connections to others are effectively fashioned and maintained? What can you do to facilitate more efficient and widespread use of this aspect of nursing practice?
5. Do you have a mentor? Why or why not? What could a mentor offer you in terms of PPM integration? How might you go about getting one?
6. How do nurses you work with notice the contributions they make to patient outcomes? Provide some examples. Do these have impact for others? How might you capitalize on this?

For Nurse Leaders

1. Describe the nurse leader's responsibility to demonstrate monetary value in relation to PPM integration.
2. Discuss the importance of aligning PPM integration with business goals. Name two or three business goals that demonstrate such alignment. What metrics would you use to assess these? Be specific.
3. Of the methods described in this chapter to link demonstration outputs with others, which one do you prefer? Why? Is there another that might be beneficial? How would you go about establishing such methods?
4. What would it take to *apply* outputs regarding PPM integration at your health system into other systems? Why? How could you be influential in this process?
5. Name three ways you use scanning to identify upcoming risks and opportunities in nursing or health care? How could you better facilitate such business tactics? Can you identify someone in the organization whom you could work with on this?
6. Explain the difference between *dissemination* and *impact*.
7. List at least three powerful consequences of PPM integration that would demonstrate value to stakeholders. How could you facilitate their attainment in your system? Be specific.

8. Do you have a mentor? Why or why not? Could you use one? How would you find a mentor to engage with you on PPMs? How would you know if the mentorship worked?

9. What assumptions about the future do you regularly analyze? Why or why not? What are your findings?

10. Describe how your health system connects with others to learn and progress. How effective are those systems? How do you know? How efficient are they? How do you know? How could you revise these systems to improve effectiveness and efficiency? Or could you? Why?

11. What stakeholder forums do you regularly participate in? Why or why not? Are they effective? What can you do to increase stakeholder engagement?

12. How do you notice nursing's contributions to the bottom line? What do you do with this information?

For Nurse Educators

1. What learning activities could best help undergraduate students understand the concept of *impact*? Why is this important for them to understand? What about graduate students?

2. What evidence is available about impact to help you best explain its importance? How might this apply to your current curriculum?

3. Develop at least three objectives for a learning activity focused on impact. What evaluation methods will you use to ensure its comprehension and application?

4. Develop a learning activity on the types of impact to help students better understand its nature. In what program or level do you see its relevance? How could this learning activity be revised for nurse leaders?

5. How might you best help students learn about ROI? Include ways to translate clinical benefits into dollars. Be specific.

6. What specific experiences would help students learn to differentiate dissemination practices from impact? How might these be used by faculty to enhance learning by students?

7. What impact is generated by your programs? Are they applied widely? What about the efficiency of application? How do you personally link with other educators to advance the positive consequences of your programs?

8. How often does your school or program examine assumptions about nursing or health systems of the future? Why or why not? How might this activity facilitate program planning?

9. How is mentorship used in your organization? Explain. Does it work? How could the process be changed to take more advantage of mentoring activities? Do you know?

10. What methods are used by your organization to connect with others for the purposes of applying lessons learned and best practices or translating research findings? If none, what could you do to advance one?

11. Who are the relevant stakeholders in your institution? What stakeholder forums do you regularly participate in? Why or why not? Are they effective? What can you do to increase stakeholder engagement? Why is this important?

12. How do you encourage students and other educators to "notice" nursing's value?

LEARNING FROM THE FIELD: IMPACT OF A LIVING PROFESSIONAL PRACTICE MODEL ON A PATIENT'S QUESTION—"HOW LONG WOULD IT TAKE TO DIE?"

Ask any nurse at Moffitt Cancer Center (MCC) about her or his patients, and she or he will say they are special. Walking through the halls with the eyes of a nurse and having the privilege of being at the bedside/chairside is a humbling and life-changing experience; however, it is also inspiring.

The faces of patients and families navigating a journey that is beyond words reflect courage, strength, fear, determination, and sometimes, loss of hope. It is evident that nurses recognize the honor and privilege of being allowed into the lives of patients and families during their most vulnerable time. They are keenly aware of the myriad of emotions and special needs as they focus on providing quality patient care. Considering all of the factors involved in caring for these "special" patients, one has to wonder how a Moffitt nurse knows what "impact she or he makes" and what that looks and feels like in real life?

The professional practice model (PPM) at MCC provides a synergistic framework for how nurses deliver care. Patients and families are the heartbeat of this model, which is strengthened by shared decision making, highlighting the value of the nurse's voice. Distinct nursing values that resonate with the art and science of nursing and align with the PPM further support how care is delivered and empower nurses to make evidence-based decisions that positively impact patient outcomes. The PPM is a living document described by one nurse as "the perfect way to put into words and pictures what nurses do every day."

Chantel's story reflects the PPM in the everyday life of a nurse caring for a patient with cancer. Initially, she did not think her caring story was a big deal...you decide.

I cared for this patient for 3 nights. The first night, her mucositis was so bad that I worried about her airway. I had her on oxygen all night, and her pain was so intense that she struggled to swallow. The second night was better and, by the third night, her mucositis was improving, oxygen was not needed, and she could swallow; however, she started to develop problems that caused additional pain. I could tell that she was feeling discouraged, and around midnight she asked, "How long would it take?" I responded, "How long would what take?" and she said, "To die, if I stopped and refused everything, how long would it take?" At this point, I said, "Let's talk...."

I sat down on her bed, held her hands, and stayed with her for over an hour. I tried to help her see the progress she had made over the past 3 nights and reminded her how strong she had become and how much her mucositis had improved. She hadn't realized the progress she had made and was grateful for my reminders. I then explained what it would be like if she refused treatment. She smiled through her tears and nodded "yes" when I asked if she felt better about making her decision.

As I started to walk out of the room, she thanked me for everything. I don't really know if she remembers me or that night, but it's a night I will never forget. The meaningful PPM that grounds our practice, our system's visionary leadership, and the engagement of nurses passionate about providing excellent care continue to make a difference for our "special" patients every day. But, the impact this patient made on me in terms of how precious nursing really is, how it influences my life for the better, and how it demonstrates to me over and over again the privilege I have to engage with such courageous persons on a daily basis, is profound.

Pamela Duncan
Chantel Fusco

REFERENCES

American Association of Colleges of Nursing (AACN). (1990). *Resolution: Need for collaborative relationships between nursing education and practice.* Washington, DC: Author.

Baumbusch, J. L., Kirkham, S. R., Khan, K. B., McDonald, H., Semeniuk, P., Tan, E., & Anderson, J. M. (2008). Pursuing common agendas: A collaborative model for knowledge translation between research and practice in clinical settings. *Research in Nursing & Health, 31*(2), 130–140.

Beal, J. A. (2012). Academic-service partnerships in nursing: An integrative review. *Nursing Research and Practice, 2012*, 1–9. doi:10.1155/2012/501564

Buxton, M., & Hanney, S. (1996). How can payback from health services research be assessed? *Journal of Health Service Research and Policy, 1*(1), 35–43.

Buzachero, V. V., Phillips, J., Phillips, P. P., & Phillips, Z. L. (2013). *Measuring ROI in healthcare*. New York, NY: McGraw-Hill.

Chandler, C. (2014). What is the meaning of impact in relation to research and why does it matter? A view from inside academia. In P. Denicolo (Ed.), *Achieving impact in research* (pp. 1–9). Los Angeles, CA: Sage.

Cheung, R. B., Aiken, L. H., Clarke, S. P., & Sloane, D. M. (2008). Nursing care and patient outcomes: International evidence. *Enfermeria Clinica, 18*(1), 35–40.

Economic and Social Research Council. (2015). *What is impact?* Retrieved March 15, 2015, from http://www.esrc.ac.uk/funding-and-guidance/impact-toolkit/what-how-and-why/what-is-research-impact.aspx

Gagliardi, A. R., Perrier, L., Webster, F., Leslie, K., Bell, M., Levinson, W., . . . Straus, S. E. (2009). Exploring mentorship as a strategy to build capacity for knowledge translation research and practice: Protocol for a qualitative study. *Implementation Science, 4,* 55. doi:10.1186/1748-5908-4-55

Gale, S. A., & Beal, J. A. (2013). Building academic-practice partnerships: Sharing best practices. *Nurse Leader, 11,* 21–24.

Karcher, M. J., Kuperminc, G. P., Portwood, S. G., Sipe, C. L., & Taylor, A. S. (2006). Mentoring programs: A framework to inform program development, research, and evaluation. *Journal of Community Psychology, 34*(6), 709–725.

Kutney-Lee, A., McHugh, M. D., Sloane, D. M., Cimiotti, J. P., Flynn, L., Neff, D. F., & Aiken, L. H. (2009). Nursing: A key to patient satisfaction. *Health Affairs (Millwood), 28*(4), w669–w677. doi:10.1377/hlthaff.28.4.w669

Lavis, J. N., Robertson, D., Woodside, J. M., McLeod, C. B., & Abelson, J. (2003). How can research organizations more effectively transfer research knowledge to decision makers? *Milbank Quarterly, 81*(2), 221–248.

Pablos-Mendez, A., & Shademani, R. (2006). Knowledge translation in global health. *Journal of Continuing Education in the Health Professions, 26*(1), 81–86.

Pittman, P., Bass, E., & Hargraves, J. (2015). Developing leadership talent: A statewide nurse leader mentorship program. *Journal of Nursing Administration, 45*(3), 63–66.

Smith, S., Shochet, R., Keeley, M., Fleming, A., & Moynahan, K. (2014). The growth of learning communities in undergraduate medical education. *Academic Medicine, 89*(6), 928–933.

Williamson, K., Almaskari, M., Lester, Z., & Maguire, D. (2015). Utilization of evidence-based practice knowledge, attitude, and skill of clinical nurses in the planning of professional development programming. *Journal for Nurses in Professional Development, 31*(2), 73–80.

Woolf, S. H., Purnell, J. Q., Simon, S. M., Zimmerman, E. B., Camberos, G. J., Haley, A., & Fields, R. P. (2015). Translating evidence into population health improvement: Strategies and barriers. *Annual Review of Public Health, 36,* 463–482.

Afterword

In most health systems today, numerous new initiatives are implemented (almost hourly); so many, that health professionals often refer to them as the flavors of the week. Sometimes there is insufficient evidence that these new approaches will work and nurses anticipate uncertain futures, fear of disruptions in workflow, and often experience general unease. Alternatively, nurse leaders frequently see similar faces doing all the work, experience pressure from above for immediate results, and encounter the all-too-familiar staff complacency. Some practice changes inevitably occur, but the intended outcomes often do not materialize quickly enough or penetrate thoroughly. In fact, many health professionals quickly drift back into their old habits, clinging to what is known, and stalling the process. Often, this results in loss of precious resources, image, and even market share. In a world with limited resources, this familiar scenario simply cannot be sustained.

Change represents something different—it is uncomfortable, scary, and downright painful at times. In complex health systems with multiple hierarchical levels, rules-based leaders, and short-term thinking, introducing something new, when the expectation for behavior change is high, is always complicated. And, if the change is connected only at the cognitive level, it may never be fully integrated.

In nursing, professional practice models (PPMs) offer a way to think about nursing practice based on disciplinary values, linking practice with values as well as intellect. Energized by direct care nurses who are passionate in their beliefs about nursing and empowered by mutually dynamic relationships with nurse leaders, integrating PPMs provides a shared purpose that combines the best and most enduring nursing principles with modern health care realities.

When driven by direct care nurses, PPMs align feelings with thoughts and actions, generating a force powerful enough to counteract old habits. Through a series of systematic phases from design to generating impact, successful integration of PPMs may provide the compelling motivation for outstanding and reliable professional nursing practice that meets the unique needs of individuals and families.

The integration process outlined in this text provides an opportunity to rethink how change, especially practice change, is implemented, evaluated, adapted, enculturated, sustained, and disseminated in nursing. In doing so, it unknowingly creates the foundation for a more systematic, evidence-based approach that may provide direction for any large-scale change. Moreover, the emphasis on evidence—its generation and use, accountability, and relationships—may translate into lasting organizational behaviors not necessarily related to integration of the PPM. Finally, demonstrating the impact of PPMs reveals the significant contributions nurses make to patients, the discipline, and their health systems.

Although many organizations have expended great resources on professional practice implementation, little is known about *how* they are implemented, whether they are consistently evaluated and with what metrics, or what specifically nurses do differently in these settings that contributes to safe, high-quality, patient-centered, efficient, and equitable care. Although some have disseminated lessons learned or best practices about PPM implementation, little high-quality evidence has been produced, and the translation of this work into clinical practice in multiple populations and sites has not been maximized. Furthermore, the differences nursing PPMs make in terms of positively impacting patient outcomes, including the health of communities, health system costs, and meaningful work for nurses are lacking, limiting nursing's ability to demonstrate their contributions.

Without demonstrating the impact of nursing PPMs, their widespread uptake in real-world practice settings is limited. A renewed emphasis on the "so what" factor regarding PPMs is desperately needed among nurse leaders, nurse researchers, clinicians, educators, health care systems, and policy makers. Demonstration of the *outcomes* produced, specifically improving patient safety and quality, health system costs, and meaningful work for nurses, must become a reality. The following strategies may help exhibit PPMs' impact:

- Conduct rigorous evaluation studies of PPMs that include the measurement of outcomes of importance to patients, nursing, and health systems.
- Conduct pilot studies that compare PPM-guided nursing care with usual nursing care.
- Prepare the next generation of nurses and nurse leaders to assume accountability for documenting the outcomes from PPM integration.

- Discourage past practices from interfering with current strategies.
- Form partnerships with academia to facilitate methodological and publication skills, speeding up the dissemination and spread of evidence about PPMs.
- Accelerate the use of analytical software among nurses and nurse leaders.
- Build environments of transparency and "safe space" within health systems to allow for increased innovation.

Nursing is notorious for proposing solutions for improving health care. However, strong data (evidence) for practice changes are necessary to showcase what and how nursing contributes to health care. With the documentation of key outcomes that health systems currently value, PPM integration will be more visible, drive responses, and generate stakeholder value that will be impossible not to acknowledge.

Such a process requires leadership, both clinical leadership and system leadership, that collaboratively creates a vision, offers a steady structure, and mobilizes the workforce through empowering and enabling behaviors while ensuring that the PPM stays aligned with the organizational mission. Nurse leaders, who model "how to be in relationship" with others and who pay relentless attention to professional nursing practice, inspire imitation. Forward-looking attitudes open to both internal and external sources—external speakers, internal evaluators, visits with other sites, selective hiring, and innovative suggestions—encourage new ways of being and doing.

Clinical nurses (ideally a cross-section of the health system) who "get" it (about professional nursing practice), who are creative and work together with leadership to enculturate a way of practice that is passionate, caring, and empowering are needed to motivate and activate others. These two forces—one steady and calming, the other creative and trailblazing—offer the persuasive, relational approach needed for successful integration.

Example: Values Clarification Workshop

DESCRIPTION

An organizational reflective process for uncovering/rediscovering the values inherent in nursing

FACILITATOR

To be announced

OBJECTIVES

By the conclusion of this activity, the participants will be able to:

1. Increase awareness of their own beliefs pertinent to nursing
2. Generate a list of core values relevant to nursing practice
3. Determine congruency between personal beliefs about nursing and health system nursing practice
4. Create a written nursing philosophy statement based on articulated nursing values

RESOURCES REQUIRED

Classroom space, audio–visual equipment, wall boards, paper, and markers

LEARNING STRATEGIES

Group discussion, reflection, group facilitation techniques, and appropriate analytical methods

EVALUATION

Formative Evaluation

Attainment of specific program/course objectives

Summative Evaluation

Nurse satisfaction with the sessions; documented nursing philosophy statement

Example: Implementation Booster Sessions

DESCRIPTION

These activities are designed to reinforce, advance, and sustain the knowledge, skills, and attitudes crucial to the professional practice model and provide opportunities for personal and professional growth.

FACULTY

To be announced

RESOURCES REQUIRED

Classrooms and audio–visual equipment, sign-in sheets, and electronic media

LEARNING STRATEGIES

Multiple forms of learning will be offered in order to accommodate individual learning styles, personal preferences, and special circumstances. Specifically, in-person lectures, videos, electronic independent study modules, study groups and learning camps, reflection seminars, and formal "sabbaticals" may be used. The program, developed in collaboration with the implementation task force of the Nursing Education Department, will be offered continuously onsite according to a regular schedule (to be determined) at convenient times for the staff. Contact hours will be awarded.

OBJECTIVES

By the conclusion of this activity, the participants will be able to:

1. State the major concepts of the professional practice model
2. Appraise their own practice in relation to the professional practice model
3. Maintain integrity to the professional practice model
4. Activate new behaviors pertinent to the professional practice model

EVALUATION

Formative Evaluation

Attainment of specific session objectives

Summative Evaluation

Evaluation of the session; observation of clinical behaviors

Example: Organizational Assessment of Professional Practice Model Integration

Indicators	Not Met	Needs Improvement	Met	Supporting Evidence
Organization's (or division of nursing's) strategic plan reflects the professional practice model				
Policy statements and procedural instructions promote the professional practice model				
The nursing strategic plan is revisited annually and adapted based on evidence				
Nursing practice decision-making processes and procedures consider the professional practice model				
Health system committees have an equitable representation of nurses who can articulate the professional practice model				
Nursing governance current bylaws reflect the professional practice model				
Attendance at governance meetings is consistently high (> 80%)				

(continued)

(continued)

Indicators	Not Met	Needs Improvement	Met	Supporting Evidence
Coordination among nursing departments is consistent with the professional practice model				
A formal recognition system for exemplary professional practice is evident				
Sufficient financial resources are allocated to professional practice model integration (including evaluation, dissemination)				
Evaluation of the professional practice model is ongoing				
The professional practice model evaluation plan reflects an appropriate mix of quantitative and qualitative data collection is used				
Health system uses professional practice model evaluation data in future planning				
Accurate and timely dissemination of professional practice model information/ materials/feedback is evident in all clinical departments				
Timely dissemination of professional practice model lessons learned and best practices is evident				
Organization is strategic about improving enculturation of the professional practice model				
The defined patient care delivery system is well aligned with the stated professional practice model				
Overall employee norms of behavior reflect the professional practice model				
Regular environmental scans and networking are used to identify and benchmark health systems with similar professional practice models				

(continued)

(continued)

Indicators	Not Met	Needs Improvement	Met	Supporting Evidence
RN job descriptions include expectations for the professional practice model				
Hiring, advancement, and professional development decisions are made in light of the "fit" with the professional practice model				
RNs provide care in a way that best utilizes their full scope of practice and spectrum of competencies				
New-employee orientation is based on the professional practice model				
The system for performance appraisal includes components of the professional practice model				
Employees are comfortable expressing their opinions and report "feeling heard"				
Employee performance reviews provide an opportunity to reflect on professional practice				
Nurse leaders set clear expectations for professional practice (consistent with the professional practice model)				
Nurse leaders understand and can inform others about all components of the professional practice model				
Nurse leaders assume accountability for ongoing support and development of professional nursing practice				
Nurse leaders exemplify the professional practice model				
Nurse leaders are transparent in their communications about professional practice				
Clinical unit leaders champion the professional practice model				

(continued)

(continued)

Indicators	Not Met	Needs Improvement	Met	Supporting Evidence
Nurse leaders regularly recognize excellent professional practice				
Nurse leaders ensure the congruence of the care delivery system and the professional practice model				
Nurse leaders facilitate evaluation and dissemination of professional practice model outcomes				
Nurse leaders provide "safe space" for employees to provide feedback				
Nurse leaders facilitate research and evidence-based practice				
There is an established succession plan to ensure sustained professional practice (consistent with the professional practice model)				
Faculty members who teach clinical courses in the health system are aware of the professional practice model and adhere to it during clinical teaching and learning				
Orientation preceptors possess the requisite competencies for practice consistent with the professional practice model				
Dedicated professional practice model educational resources are available (to all employees regardless of shifts worked) to support ongoing learning				
Educational offerings related to the professional practice model use various interactive teaching strategies and evaluation mechanisms				
Unit artifacts are welcoming, informative, and consistent with the professional practice model				

(continued)

(continued)

Indicators	Not Met	Needs Improvement	Met	Supporting Evidence
Nurses and other employees can describe features of the professional practice model				
Nurses and other employees can relay how the professional practice model is operationalized on the unit				
There is evidence of professional practice model language in the medical record				
Employees state they are confident in their ability to perform the professional practice model				
RNs assume accountability for exemplary professional practice				
The professional practice model is perceived as compatible with RN work				
Evidence of employee motivation (goal-oriented behaviors) to practice within the professional practice model is apparent				

IMPROVEMENT PLAN

_____

_____

_____

_____

_____

_____

_____

_____

_____

_____

Index

Abelson, J., 264
accountability, 103–105, 199–201.
　　See also professional practice
　　models (PPM)
　　for "living," 11
　　professional, 138
accountability-based system, 64
accountable care organizations
　　(ACOs), 8
adapting implementation strategies,
　　153–160. *See also* implementation
　　of professional practice model
　　balancing action and reflection for
　　　rapid integration, 162–165
　　engaging clinical microsystems,
　　　160–161
　　implementation committees, role of,
　　　155–157
　　leadership implications, 158–159
　　organizational factors, 157–159
　　Texas Health Resources (THR), case
　　　of, 168–169
*A Data Driven Approach to Nurse
　　Engagement: Key Insights and Best
　　Practices from the Experts*, 201
adoption of professional practice models
　　individual, 173–178
　　meaningful (or meaningless) work
　　　environments, 181–182
　　milestones, 179–180
　　tipping points, 178–179

Advisory Board Company, 201
Advocate Health System in Illinois,
　　52–53, 252–254
Affordable Care Act, 30
Agency for Healthcare Research and
　　Quality (AHRQ), 127
alignment with professional practice
　　model, 191–201. *See also* adoption
　　of professional practice models;
　　implementation of professional
　　practice model
American Nurses Credentialing
　　Center (ANCC) Magnet®
　　criteria, 64
American Nurses Association (ANA)
　　Code of Ethics, 50
Aplin, L., 237
Attending Nurse Model, 8
Attending Physician Model, 8
authentic leadership, 105.
　　See also leadership

Bass, E., 265
Bate, P., 173
being professional, 36
best practices, 235–237
big data, 264
*Blueprint for 21st Century Nursing Ethics:
　　Report of the National Nursing
　　Summit*, 37
body sensors, 264

career advancement systems, 9

career ladders, 9

Cleland, V. S., 9

clinical advancement programs
    (or clinical ladders), 68

clinical microsystems, 161

clinical workflow, 93–95. *See also*
    implementation of professional
    practice model; professional
    practice models (PPM)

coaching, 97

collaborative peer group, 164

Colquhoun, A., 237

commitment, 39–41

communication strategies for
    professional practice model,
    95–96

compatibility, 240

competencies for professional practice,
    198–199

  generic, 198

  technical, 199

Context, Inputs, Process, and Product
    (CIPP) evaluation framework,
    124

continuum of care, 24

control group design, 102

convenience sampling, 131

costs of professional practice model
    integration, 29–31

  direct, 30

  indirect, 30

  maintenance, 30

  opportunity, 30

Creating Authentic Relationships
    Everyday (CARE), 109–110

creative patient-centered solutions, 21

DAISY award, 10

decision-making process, 155

Delphi technique, 52

Denis, J. L., 224

developmental feedback, 98

DiClemente, C. C., 174

Diffusion of Innovation Theory, 175, 179

Dik, B. J., 181

dissemination of lessons learned and
    best practices, 237–240

  in Advocate Health System in Illinois,
    252

  ExpandNet/WHO framework for
    scaling up, 242

  frameworks and methods of
    distribution, 240–245

  Institute for Healthcare
    Improvement's (IHI) evolving
    Framework for Spread, 241

  leadership and, 245–248

  methods of distribution, 243–245

  PCORI Dissemination and
    Implementation Framework, 242,
    245

  University of Washington Health
    Promotion Research Center
    (HPRC) framework, 241

  Value-Added Research Dissemination
    Framework, 241–242

Dynamic Sustainability Framework
    (DSF), 218

Edmundson, E., 56

emotional intelligence, 20

empowerment

  clinicians, 94

  nurses, 23, 64, 209

  others, 38, 96, 98, 145

enculturation, health system, 189–191

end-of-project outcomes reports, 125

epidemics, 178

evaluation, 115–120. *See also* evaluation
    methods

  of Centers for Disease Control and
    Prevention's (CDC) program,
    123–124

Context, Inputs, Process, and Product (CIPP) evaluation framework, 124
data for, 118, 126–129
engaging stakeholders in, 136
formative, 116–117
framework for professional practice model, 120–125
goal of, 116
goal-free, 121–122
goals-based (GBE), 121–122
graphical data displays, 135, 145–149
operational definition, 116
quantitative and qualitative indicators, 126
reporting of results, 134–137
selecting a logical indicator set for, 125–126
summative, 116–117
timing of, 135
value of systemic, 137–140
visual representation of data, 135
evaluation methods
data analysis, 132–133
data collection, 129–130
human subjects, 130
interpretation of results, 133
sampling, 130–132
evidence-based implementation strategies, 101
evidence-based practice (EBP), 9, 54
external evidence, 26–27
external integration, 24. *See also* integration

facilitator, 51
feedback on professional practice model, 97–99
developmental, 98
effective, 98
good, 99
overloading on, 99

Fleiszer, A. R., 224
Fong, K. T., 38
forecasting, 264
formal recognition, 68. *See also* recognition programs
formative evaluation, 116–117, 154, 278, 280. *See also* evaluation
functional nursing, 8

Gagliardi, A. R., 263
gaps in nursing practice, analysis of, 28–29
Geary, J., 237
generalizability, 132
Generating and Assessing Evidence for Nursing Practice, 9th Edition, 129
generic competencies, 198–199
Gladwell, Malcolm
  The Tipping Point: How Little Things Can Make a Big Difference, 178, 241
goal statement, 122
goal-free evaluation (GFE), 121–122. *See also* evaluation
goals-based evaluation (GBE), 121–122. *See also* evaluation
Goldsmith, M., 64
Goodman, K. J., 237
governance in health care delivery, 63–66
Greenhalgh, T., 173
guiding principles, 59–60

Hargraves, J., 265
Hatcher, J., 237
health care directories, 265
health system enculturation, 189–191
Hoebel, E. A., 190
Hoffart, N., 4
holistic care, 21
Hospital Consumer Assessment of Healthcare Providers and Systems (HCAHPS), 107, 126

impact of PPM, 257–258
 actualizing future, 264–265
 high, 261–264
 at Moffitt Cancer Center (MCC),
  269–270
 nature of, 259–261
implementation of professional
  practice model. *See also* adapting
  implementation strategies;
  professional practice models
  (PPM)
 accountability and, 103–105
 action-oriented learning activities,
  89
 chief nurse executive, role of, 107–109
 coaching, 97
 criteria for selecting strategies, 88
 designing booster strategies, 99–101,
  279–280
 education and training for, 88–90
 effective communication, 95–96
 encouragement and reinforcement, 96
 evidence-based, 101
 graduated approach, 102
 implementation plan, 79–86, 164
 implementation strategies, 86–101
 innovative strategies, 109–110
 modes of implementation, 101–103
 modifying work roles and
  responsibilities, 90–93
 providing feedback, 97–99
 redesigning clinical workflow, 93–95
 role delineation, 90–91
 safe space, creating, 96–97
 systematic implementation
  approaches, 102
 template, 104
 unit-level formative data for, 143–145
 whole-system start-up, 101
Indiana University Health, 5
Indiana University Health's mission, 5–6
indicators

 qualitative, 126
 quantitative, 126
individual nursing characteristics, 20
Institute of Medicine (IOM) *Future of*
  Nursing report, 38
integration
 commitment in the context of, 40
 costs of, professional practice models,
  29–31
 defined, 24
 external, 24
 internal, 24
 organizational assessment of, 281–286
 preintegration, 25–31
 preparing, for professional practice
  models, 26
 of professional practice models,
  24–25
internal evidence, 27–28
internal integration, 24. *See also*
  integration
interprofessional collaboration, 37
interprofessionalism, 37–38
interprofessional teamwork, 37–38

Kahn, W. A., 201
knowledgeable consultants, 265
knowledge transfer, 243–244, 248, 262
Kotter, J. P., 26, 223
Kotter and Rathgeber's change model,
  108, 223
Kyriakidou, O., 173

Lavis, J. N., 264
leadership, 38–39, 97
 authentic, 105
 dissemination of lessons learned and
  best practices and, 245–248
 as a lifelong process, 39
 position-based, 63–64
 shared, 63–66
 transformational, 38–39

learning organizations, 165
lessons learned and best practices,
    235–237
dissemination of, 237–240
Level of Institutionalization Scales
    (LoIn) of health promotion
    programs, 221–222
licensed practical nurse (LPN), 57
Lips-Wiersma, M., 181
Lowell General Hospital, 53–54

MacFarlane, F., 173
Magnet®, 208
    criterion of structural
        empowerment, 8
    gap analysis tool, 28
Management Systems International
    (MSI), 239
Mancini, J. A., 222
Marek, L. I., 222
Mazzocco, K., 38
McLeod, C. B., 264
MD Anderson Nursing Professional
    Practice Model, 73–74
meaningful recognition, 66–67. *See also*
    recognition programs
milestones, 179–180
mission statement of an organization,
    4–5, 53–55
Moffitt Cancer Center (MCC), 269–270

National Database of Nursing Quality
    Indicators (NDNQI), 127
Nine Steps for Developing a Scaling-up
    Strategy, 240
Nonpartnered Clinical Model, 8
Norcross, J. C., 174
Novant Health Prince William Medical
    Center (NHPWMC), 145–149
    attentive reassurance and healing
        environment, 146
    critical care unit, 149

nurse–patient relationships at, 148
    outpatient services, 147–148
    plan of care for post-operative
        patients, 146
    urinary catheter removal, 146
nursing case management, 57
nursing practice, organizational
    expression of, 22. *See also*
    professional nursing practice
Nursing Quality Indicators (NDNQI),
    127
Nursing Research: Generating and
    Assessing Evidence for Nursing
    Practice, 129
nursing's contribution to health care, 3
Nursing's Social Policy Statement, 35
nursing values, 49–53
    consistency between mission
        statement and, 54–55

onboarding, 196–197
optimal nurse staffing plans, 61
Orem's self-care theory, 100
organizational characteristics, 7
organizational expression of nursing
    practice, 22
organizational memory, 219–221
organizational missions, 53–56
Organizational Readiness to Change
    Assessment (ORCA), 28
organization-sponsored networking
    events, 68

PARiHS framework, 177
Partnered Model, 8
patient care delivery system (PCDS), 4,
    6–8, 57–62
    activities used to design a, 59
    developing, 73–74
    traditional, 8
patient-centered medical homes
    (PCMH), 8

Patient-Centered Outcomes Research
    Institute (PCORI), 238
PCORI Dissemination and
    Implementation Framework,
    242–245
personalized medicine, 264
Pettiti, D. B., 38
Pittman, P., 265
point-of-care diagnostics, 264
Porter-O'Grady, T., 9
positive reinforcement, 96
primary data, 126–127
primary nursing, 8
primary team nursing (PTN), 73–74
printing of organs, 264
private duty nursing, 8
probability sampling, 131
Prochaska, J. O., 174
professional accountability, 138
professionalism, 21
professional journals, 265
professional nursing practice, 43–44
    individual nursing characteristics, 20
    patient-centered solutions, 21
    realities of, 19–22
professional practice models (PPM),
    50, 59, 65, 67–69, 220. See also
    sustainability of PPMs
    accountability, 199–201
    competencies required for, 198–199
    components of, 4–10
    defined, 3–4, 12
    definition of professional nursing, 62
    developing, 73–74
    hiring practices and, 193–195
    impact of (see impact of PPM)
    implications of, 10–12
    inclusion, 56
    integration, process of, 24–25, 54–55,
        138
    living the, 201–203
    nurse engagement, 200–201

onboarding, 196–197
philosophical statements
    supporting, 5
professional values of, 73–74
progression of, 192
specialty's recommendations for,
    15–16
talent development, 197–198
ultimate goal of, 4
value of, 22–24, 32–33
visual representation, 4
professional values, 3, 22–23, 73–74
Program Evaluation Standards, 119
Program Sustainability Assessment Tool
    (PSAT), 221
Program Sustainability Index (PSI), 222
public health discipline and
    sustainability, 216–219

Quality-Caring Model© (QCM), 6, 73, 92,
    107, 145, 171, 228
    eight caring factors of, 73–74
    individual adoption of, 185–186

random sampling, 131
reach, effectiveness, adoption,
    implementation, maintain
    (RE-AIM) method, 119
recognition programs, 66–69
    formal, 68
    informal, 68
    meaningful, 66–67
registered nurses (RN), 3–4, 8, 89–90, 190
    as associates, 8
    24-hour accountability for patient
        care, 8
reinforcement, 96
reliability, 127–128
remotely delivered health care, 264
rewarding professional nurses, 66–69
Richer, M., 224

Ritchie, J. A., 224
Robert, G., 173
Robertson, D., 264
Rogers, E. M., 175, 179
role delineation, 90–91
   information collected during, 91
Rosso and colleagues, 181
routinization cycles, 217, 222

safe space, creating, 96–97
Scalability Assessment Tool (SAT)
   checklist, 240
scaling up, 238–239
scanning and monitoring, 264
Schaufeli, W. B., 200
Scheirer, M. A., 223
Schell, S. F., 216
secondary data, 127
self-control, 176
Semenic, S. E., 224
Senge, P. M., 165
   Dance of Change, 26
sexual assault nurse examiners (SANEs),
   15–16
shared governance, 9
shared governance systems, 65–66
   designing of, 65
   examples of activities in, 66
shared leadership, 63–66. *See also*
   leadership
   benefits of, 64
shared work-related values, 50
social cognitive theory (SCT), 174
socializing or resocializing nurses,
   190
social learning theory (SLT), 174
social network theory or social network
   analysis (SNA), 176–177
stakeholders, role in evaluation, 136
Steger, M. F., 181
Stein, E. W., 219
Stirman, S. W., 222

strengths, weaknesses, and
   opportunities/threats (SWOT)
   analysis, 82–84
summative evaluation, 116–117, 119, 278,
   280. *See also* evaluation
Surgical Care Improvement Project
   (SCIP), 146
sustainability of PPMs. *See also*
   professional practice models
   (PPM)
   delegating, 228
   developing, 227–232
   enhancing, 223–224
   frameworks, 216–221
   innovative approaches, 231–232
   key documents and programs for,
      228–230
   leadership support, 230–231
   measuring, 221–222
   nature of, 215–216
   nurse rewards for, 231
   of SANE programs, 15–16
Synergy Model, 6
systematic assessment, 118
systematic sampling, 131

talent development, 197–198, 203
team nursing, 8
technical competencies, 199
Texas Health Arlington Memorial
   Hospital (THAM), 208–209
Texas Health Resources (THR), 168–171
   "Healing Hands. Caring Hearts"
      slogan, 208
   pain management initiative, 170
   professional development, 170–171
   professional practice model, 169–171
   Quality-Caring Model©, 171
   shared decision making, 171
   teamwork, 170
theoretical foundation of nursing
   practice, 55–56

theory of planned behavior (TPB), 176
theory of reasoned action, 176
tipping points, 178–179
total patient care, 8
transferability of nurses' clinical
    skills, 189, 190
transformational leadership, 38, 39
Transforming Care at the Bedside
    (TCAB) initiative, 94
transparency, 136–137
transtheoretical model, 174, 182
trialability, 240
t-test, 133

*Understanding Nursing Research: Building
    an Evidence-based Practice*, 129
Ungson, G. R., 219
University of California San Diego
    (UCSD) Health System, 4–5

University of Washington Health
    Promotion Research Center
    (HPRC) framework, 241
unlicensed assistive personnel (UAP), 57

validity, 127–128
Value-Added Research Dissemination
    Framework, 241–242

Walsh, J. P., 219
Watson's caring theory, 62
whole-system start-up, 101
Wisdom, J. P., 177
Woods, C. Q., 4
Woodside, J. M., 264
work engagement, 200–201
Wright, S., 181

Yin's Routinization Framework, 217

Printed in the United States
By Bookmasters